Diet Like a Guru

It's What You Put in Your Heart – Not in Your Tummy

By

Dr. Rosie Kuhn

Table of Contents

Introduction

Diet like a guru! Really?

"*Diet*", to many of us, is a four-letter word. Immediately we imagine deprivation, emotionality, and ways to put off until tomorrow any activity that requires change, challenge, and hard work.

There is another way to attend to our well-being – No deprivation required! This way is different than other weight-loss, or diet processes in that it empowers you to explore with curiosity your relationship with yourself. It is only with yourself that the conversations about food and what it will give you occurs. When you uncover your specific beliefs and interpretations in relation to food, drinks, and all substances, you instantly have access to free choice. And, if what you want is to thrive in well-being, it might make sense to look at the mechanisms that are interfering with you having what you want. That makes sense, right?

Gurus Don't Diet

Yes, gurus don't diet. They don't use substances to mask or numb themselves from emotional pain and fears either. They empower themselves to look at their emotions, thoughts, and body sensations mindfully. With presence of mind, they uncover old patterns of thinking and believing that no longer make sense, except within the unexamined vault of wounds.

You and I are no different from any guru I'm aware of. You have the same capabilities to choose in service of your highest truths and values. And every guru began where you are now – in doubt, fear, and resistance. They, like you, decided that something is more important than numbing, avoiding, and distracting their minds from their true selves, and the lives they've been given. They, like you, will have taken one step at a time, examining what has caused them to choose unsuccessful practices over and over again. You will find, as gurus have found, that every single moment reveals the truth of inner courage, conviction, strength, and love; they just had to see it and not turn away from it. I, like you, like every guru I know of, can, and will, inevitably choose love. It's just a matter of when.

This book, *Diet Like a Guru*, provides perspectives, stories, and ideas that will empower you to think differently about what you may have not been thinking about at all. It encourages you to question those principles and values that you've relied on for a lifetime, in support of your choice-making, regarding food, drinks, and any other substances that seem to give comfort and nurturance.

I Want My Freedom to Choose What I Want When I Want!

We believe that allowing ourselves to indulge our impulses comes about through free will. The fact of the matter is that free will allows us to choose to indulge or not to indulge. This book assists you in witnessing the degree to which you are actually freely choosing to indulge. You will notice how often you are choosing from some hidden control mechanisms you didn't even know was there. With curiosity, you will come to know yourself fully, and thus discover you can effortlessly choose freely, because you empower yourself to do so.

There is no pressure or timeline. There is nothing to do that you don't choose to do yourself. There are no should's and shouldn't's or do's and don'ts. What this practice does is provide you with a timeout, for just a few minutes every day, to be present and mindful to the thinking that has you choose to indulge in those impulses that take you away from what you truly desire: thriving health and well-being. You may choose to spend one day with each chapter, or one week, letting the theme seep into your being over more time. It's up to you how deeply you take in this practice.

You will find through the days and months ahead that you will connect with your wise inner-guru-self to support you in engaging in "dieting" as a spiritual practice. The guarantee is that you do not have to deprive yourself of anything, and there is no sacrifice; only the cultivation of true free will to *Diet Like a Guru*.

The most important thing is to have fun. If it isn't fun, or fun enough, you won't keep going. You will quit. I know!! I'm a quitter at heart, so if isn't fun, I quit.

You may be interested to visit the **YouTube Page: Diet Like a Guru**. There are 31 videos, less than 3 minutes long each, called *Guru Gumdrops*. These tasty morsels of wisdom will inspire you to be curious about you. Each one relates to a specific chapter in the book.

Chapter One
To Deprive Myself is Out of the Question

Let's jump right in with the most frequently-used statement of anyone wanting to change their way of being in the world: "I Don't Want to Deprive Myself!"… Okay!

#1 Rule of Diet Like a Guru is: You need not deprive yourself of ANYTHING!

So, with that said, you are now free to choose whatever it is you want. You can have as much as you want of whatever you want! You have the power and freedom to choose! YES!!!!

Now for the biggest conundrum you will face as you take on the practice of dieting like a guru: Either you are depriving yourself of your substances of choice, or you are depriving yourself of the health and vitality you want to experience in your life. It is a dilemma, and how we be with our dilemmas will help us move relatively gracefully towards our desired outcome.

Wait-You just told me that I didn't have to deprive myself of anything, right? What gives?

I have two questions for you that will be foundational to how you proceed through this practice: "What is it that you want? And, what is it that you want – enough - that you are willing to experiment with how you be with the dilemmas and conundrums facing you? How will you adventure into possibility?" Okay, that's 3 questions!

When I ask my clients these questions, they often say: "I want to be healthy; I want to lose weight; I want to bring more exercise into my life; I want to be a model of healthy living for my children; I want to be happy and fulfilled. AND… I want to continue to indulge my impulses- not deprive myself of anything." Excellent!

11

It is good to get it all out onto the table. And, knowing that you do not want to deprive yourself, and most likely will do whatever it takes not to deprive yourself, will go a long way to bringing you to the results you are looking for.

Believe it or not, that part of you who is adamant about avoiding deprivation believes it is looking out for your best interest. It operates on the premise that deprivation will lead to certain death. It doesn't want you to die, so it keeps wanting you to do whatever it takes to survive. This part of you is wise in the ways of surviving. It is not wise, however, in the ways of thriving. It doesn't understand that optimal living is what you actually came here to experience.

To diet like a guru means that we become mindful of how we think what we think. We develop a willingness to be curious about how we be in our lives, in our bodies, in our emotions, in our spirits. We notice our desire to have it all – to deprive ourselves of nothing, yet continually deprive ourselves of what can be the most valuable assets of life: health and happiness.

To diet like a guru, there is no hurry to make any changes. There's nowhere to get to – really. You are already whole. You are already amazingly beautiful, precious, and unique. You already have everything you want. The fun part is just being curious and in wonder – enough to begin to explore where you are in your own personal evolution! It's like unwrapping a beautiful package, using the utmost tenderness and care.

Just for today, notice any fears, worries and anxiousness that may arise as you begin to consider the possibility to *maybe* diet like a guru. Notice too, perhaps some excitement, wonder, and curiosity about what might transpire through this practice. If you have the desire, you may start a journal for yourself, to write down what comes to you as you take baby steps towards saying yes!

Tell yourself that there is nothing you have to deprive yourself of today. There is nothing you have to give up; there is nothing you have to change. With tenderness and care, reassure that part of yourself that is really scared of dying by deprivation that you will now be taking very good care to not have that happen.

12

It takes only a few moments a day to realize the ease of dieting like a guru. Take a deep breath and celebrate that you've chosen to come this far today. That's it!

Chapter 2
What is the Truth?

All of us have within us a wise inner-guru, who is available to us 24-7. Our inner-guru answers every question we ask with absolute truth, because that's what it is there to do, so we can live in our fullest potentiality - the most expansive life possible.

I don't know about you, but I am not always ready to listen to that truth and the wisdom that often piggybacks on truth. And, so, I forget that my inner-guru is there, and I answer my question for myself with the same old relentless patterns that don't ever work (I rarely feel the wiser by answering my own questions by myself). So, with that said, I'm going to jump into the subject of the day:

Diet and the idea of diet is an imposed set of beliefs and interpretations that come to us by way of culture, ethnicity, family traditions, and religions: they each influence what to eat, how to eat, and when to eat.

Quite often it is through imposed acculturalization that we also learn how to use foods, and other substances, to help us cope with what reality has to throw at us. Because we are immersed and enmeshed in our cultures, our responses to food and to emotions, for that matter, become automatic: An impulse arises, and we train ourselves to feed the impulse unconsciously.

We are taught and trained by our cultures and families to ignore our truths, our suffering, and the many injustices we live with, so that the cultural ways stay intact (even when it doesn't make sense to do so.). We feel powerless to do anything but ignore and numb our pain. For many of us this is required in order to maintain enough sanity to get from one day to another. I know this, not only through my own personal experience, but through my clients' sharing of what it was like to live as if the best they could expect was to hope for a better tomorrow.

We have an interesting relationship with reality: When something is experienced as hurtful, or disappointing, few of us have the opportunity to say clearly, directly and out loud: "OUCH!" We aren't allowed to express the truth of our experience. So, with our infinite wisdom, in service to survival, we learn how to mask, avoid, and ignore the sensations of hurt.

When we use food, or any substance or activity that numbs or masks our pain, we avoid the truth of our own suffering, while ensuring our survival, and the survival of our culture.

When we become conscious of these various impulses, how we've trained ourselves to eat and how to deal with emotions, we are then at choice to choose another way. We are free to discover a way that allows us to freely express ourselves in the world. I believe that this is what we came here to experience – the fulfillment of our Human-Spirit!

I realize thus far, through my own journey to well-being, that so much of our reality doesn't make sense. In fact, it is filled with insanities. Each of us is doing the very best we can do with the tools and trainings passed down through generations to survive the circumstances of our lives. For some, the insanity is too great – betrayal, violence, and abuse in all its disguises has some of us just give up, as it is often too much for our human heart to bear.

The majority of us survive. And, while many of us long for living in wholeness, peace and happiness, few of us willingly take the path to make that happen.

Those of you who are reading this, in this moment, are willingly taking the path. You are hearing the wise inner-guru tell you that it's time; that the consequences of your current choices do not support you in experiencing the fullest expression of your essential nature; and that you have the strength and courage to hear the truth and to experiment with doing some things differently.

To diet like a guru, we practice with very small experimentations, with no dramatic results expected, good, bad, or otherwise – just to see what is possible. We exercise, stretch and strengthen muscles of listening, speaking, and experiencing our truth. We become curious and daring enough to ask questions of our inner-guru, and hear the answers we know to be our highest truths.

Just for today, listen for your truth. You might want to journal or talk with someone about these truths – a coach, a therapist, a sponsor, or minister. If you feel safe, speak your truth out loud, even if it's not the truth you want to admit to others or to yourself.

When we listen for the truth, and begin to speak our truth, even when it's not what we want to hear or to say, we begin to cultivate something exceptionally important: an authentic relationship with ourselves. When we cultivate and strengthen this authentic relationship with ourselves, we nourish self-respect, self-honor, self-appreciation, and dignity. Just small incremental shifts in this direction will allow you the ability to choose to shift what has forever felt like an imposed way of being with food, drink, and other substances.

There comes a point in every person's life when the suffering is too great, and all that is left to do is to speak the truth: "I am human. I am in pain. I am ready to live another way. Empower me to choose differently."

Chapter 3
Your Fiercest Ally Lives Within

I don't know about you, but the relationship I've had with myself for decades is one of distrust and no respect.

My actions, for the majority of my life, have reflected a need to experience love from a source outside myself. Either through food, or relationship with lovers, I've ignored my true self, and lied to her regarding my motives of operating, in service to assuaging the fears of my false self - the self that is enmeshed in surviving, not thriving. I've lied to myself and other people for the majority of my life, and I didn't even know it (D.E.N.I.A.L. = Don't Even Know I Am Lying).

Because I've been ignoring, avoiding, and lying to myself forever (to the me who has emotions and values that I don't live by), there is no trust. I don't trust myself that I will tell the truth. I don't trust that I will follow through with promises I make, to myself and to others. I have no reason to trust myself, and so I don't.

If I don't trust myself, who do I turn to in support of me keeping promises? If I don't trust myself, how am I supposed to even think that I'm going to diet like a guru? It feels to me like I'm heading down just another useless rabbit-hole. I think it's time to head for the fridge! YUCK!!!

HOLD ON NOW FOR JUST ONE MOMENT!

Because this book is about shifting perspectives and interpretations about you and your reality, what would shift if you saw that part of you, that appears to be your worst enemy, as one of your greatest allies?

Take that in for a moment.

What if that part of you that is fierce and powerful, and will not give up anything, for anyone, has exactly what you need to create right-livelihood? Can you consider *that* for just a moment, *before* you open the fridge door?

That part of you that declares: "You Can't Make Me!" is very strong and powerful. She is fierce in her desire to have power and presence in the world, and more importantly, in your life! The context of food may be the only arena where she commands a sense of presence and power. She wants to be heard, honored, and respected. In doing what she is doing, she has a voice in your life. Maybe, if you begin to listen to her, she can begin to express that fierceness in ways that support both of you in moving into more generative ways of thriving and living in your fullest potential.

I know, right? This is hard on the head to consider that you can actually work with this hard-headed woman, instead of fighting and resisting her. But just for a moment, consider what would shift if you were able to witness her as truly a powerful force in your life, and bring her in as an ally. I'm serious here, not just throwing you lovely rhetoric! I mean it!

And, of course, the question begs to be asked: What needs to shift in order for this collaborative relationship to even be possible?

#2 Rule of Diet Like a Guru is: Cultivate Self-Trust. Because, when we cultivate trust, we cultivate respect. And, when we cultivate respect, we cultivate honor and appreciation. When we cultivate honor and appreciation, we become more allowing and open, more accepting and free, and inspired and creative, and, all of a sudden, we love our lives!

To diet like a guru, we look at all the various facets of our personality with fresh eyes. Rather than seeing them as dysfunctional, incompetent, pathetic losers, who are keeping us from the life we say we want, we look at each aspect of our personality as essential partners; we see them as experiencers of life, who have been ignored, and yelled at – "shut up!" We've not trusted that their particular viewpoint is trustworthy and can be respected, because it is theirs.

To diet like a guru, we begin the process of seeing these unique parts of ourselves for the unique contribution they can make to our lives. Rather than shunning them, we choose to include them as individual parts of us who have life experiences worthy of honor. YES - HONOR!

Up until now, the shunning and avoiding haven't worked. It never, ever will! So what have we got to lose by practicing trust in one's fierceness and commanding presence? Experience has proven to me that, when trusted and respected, the most shunned enemies can and will serve your highest truth and desires.

Just for today, consider the way you have been being with all the various aspects of yourself. Notice how it feels to be you, in relation to these aspects of you that you ignore and avoid. Consider that it may take some time to shift the relationship that you've had with yourself, and that it takes time to cultivate trust within yourself, just like it takes time to cultivate trust with any person you meet.

When we take time to understand that the way we operate has brought us to this moment of consciousness and wisdom, we can trust that, through conscious choice, we can make incredible shifts in our reality. I have absolutely no doubt that this is true.

Chapter 4
Nurture Yourself with Compassion

Emancipation from Your Personal Suffering

This book empowers you to emancipate yourself from your own self-created quagmire of undesired circumstances. Once you realize that it was you, in all of your radiant brilliance, who designed the way it is, for the purpose of surviving, you can come to realize too, that you have the same brilliant capability to stop yourself from actively participating in what no longer nourishes and nurtures your thriving.

It is an amazing moment of grace when you are willing to hide nothing from yourself. It is a moment of honoring and respecting the long and arduous journey you've taken as a human being. You experience, perhaps for the first time, what dignity is, and how precious your singular life has become. Peace, joy, and fulfillment will be experienced more often, as everything you've held on to, which limits their presence within your comfort zone, will be released.

Right now, you might think this is dangerous, to explore what you've hidden away. However, much like examining the contents of a storage unit, a basement, or attic, you will uncover precious treasures, which are inherently valuable to the unfolding and the evolution of you. Truly there is nothing hiding within that you will not be grateful to discover.

Because you have free will, you can delay and wait; you can numb or paralyze yourself; you can ignore, avoid and distract; and you can choose to deny your own ability to choose wisely. You can throw yourself on the ground, in a tantrum, declaring to the world: "Yes, but it's hard work!" Trust me, we all know that it is hard work, but what had you think that it would be otherwise?

23

To diet like a guru, requires reaching out for support from time to time. 12-Step Programs, weight loss systems, such as Weight Watchers or Jenny Craig, and many others are communities that support people through this process. There are coaches and therapists too, who specialize in supporting individuals who desire guidance. Spiritual guides can also support you to be present to yourself in a way that will empower you to heal your own wounds. I am here as a coach as well, and would be honored to walk alongside you as you daringly walk this sacred path of life.

To diet like a guru, this may also be a time where you begin to expand your support team to include the spiritual realms. For me, spirituality is the practice of cultivating **faith** in something greater than ourselves. It's when we begin to create a relationship with our unseen angels, guides, and perhaps loved ones who have passed. Prayer, meditation, contemplation, journaling, or just communicating verbally, or through your thoughts, can create a sense of connection you have yet to experience directly. It is well worth the practice!

Just for today, consider what you've been using to be supported in your life's journey. What has been working for you? What hasn't worked? Quite often we expect to feel supported by people we love, but the truth is, we don't always get the support we need from them, and we may need to look elsewhere for what we need.

Consider *just for today,* creating a different support system, for the specific purpose of dieting like a guru. Notice what thoughts and feelings arise that may keep you from exploring new avenues of support.

Over time, with more ease and daring, you can sit in the discomfort of this release process. You can courageously allow yourself to recognize those fears that arise, which communicates to you the potential awakening of all that you've anesthetized, for perhaps lifetimes.

Chapter 5
There is Nothing to Do But to Notice

We are generally so disconnected from ourselves that we don't even know what drives us to engage with substances (food or other) the way we do.

The more mindful and engaged we can be with actively watching our thoughts and our behavior, the greater our capacity will be to choose, with conscious intelligence, what to think, what to do, and who to be in our lives.

When beginning some new endeavor, such as to diet like a guru, many of us start out excited about the possibilities that await the arrival at our destination. However, few of us maintain that excitement for more than a couple of weeks. Many find themselves losing interest, and begin to divert their interest with previously engaging beliefs and activities. Let's eat!

All successful accomplishments require attention, study, and discipline (boy, we hate that word as much as the word DEPRIVATION, don't we?!).

To diet like a guru, it's essential to truly decide what is important enough that you would take on such a study and exercise the muscles of discipline. If there is nothing you need to deprive yourself of, and being truthful with yourself and cultivating self-trust is really all you need to practice - what is it that will stop you from fulfilling your desired outcome?

By noticing what stops you now from fulfilling your desired outcome, you can begin to perhaps think differently about these stoppers.

What has often stopped me, is when...

1. I get overwhelmed when faced with the conflicting ideas of my old patterns and the new patterns I'll be developing for myself.

25

2. I get impatient - thinking that I should be doing something that I'm not doing, so that I'll get to my goal faster.

3. I compare myself and my progress to other people and other programs that provide "Faster, Easier, Better!"

4. I don't know what to do, and I'm feeling the angst that has, in the past, always driven me to eat.

5, I get scared that I'm going to fail, and I hate feeling the self-hate and self-loathing that always accompanies failing.

6, I expect to see immediate results.

7. I think about what other people will think or decide about me.

8. I imagine who I'll be in the future, and I'm not sure that I will like that person.

9. I wonder - What's the Point?!

10, I'm not sure I'm doing it right, so I go back to doing what I know I can do right, even if it's not going to get me the results I'm desiring.

Our thoughts always either align with our highest desires, or they are an attempt to avoid an undesirable feeling.

All 10 of my stoppers point to 3 qualities of being, all of which I'm wanting to avoid - *Powerlessness, Helplessness, and Hopelessness.*

Every person I've ever known is running as fast as they can from feeling and experiencing powerless, helpless, or hopeless. And yet, because we exist as human beings, every one of us, at times, is powerless, helpless, and hopeless.

If we all experience times of powerless, helpless, and hopeless, why are we constantly doing whatever we can to look like we are so "together"? Why do we continually create strategies to avoid, ignore, and deny our P.H.H. (Powerless, Helpless, Hopeless)?

To diet like a guru, we take on a practice of studying ourselves, our behaviors, our thoughts and emotions. We notice sensations that are sourced from fear - such as anxiety, worry, guilt, angst, despair, and others.

We begin to distinguish when we are following a fear-based thought or emotion with specific behaviors that quell the fear for moments at a time. To diet like a guru, we also begin to allow ourselves our authentic feelings of sadness, anger, and many other emotions that we've labeled as bad or wrong.

Most importantly, we watch ourselves judge our thoughts, emotions, behaviors, and sensations, as bad or good, right or wrong. Remember: no emotion, thought, action, or sensation is right, wrong, good or bad. It is what we do with them that can be harmful to ourselves or to others. So we simply watch and notice our judgments.

Over time you'll be able to shift from judging to not judging. Again, judging isn't bad or wrong. It's an important ability that we cultivate. It is how we use judging.

Do I get to feel better about myself through my judging? Do I get to make someone else wrong through my judging? Does my judging distract me from what I'm wanting to avoid or ignore that is going on inside of me?

Just for today, decide what you'd like to bring your attention to - what would you like to study about yourself? Then, throughout your day, just notice you being you. Take notes and journal if you'd find this helpful. You are investigating your self, your reality, and the way to bring about the reality you really want to enjoy. Again, just notice. *And, if you want to do something different, empower yourself to experiment. See what the results are of that experiment. You can do it again, if you'd like, or experiment with something else. Only if you want!*

28

Chapter 6
You Have Already Started

You've been preparing yourself for this moment, perhaps for a lifetime. You've been mindful and conscious of what it feels like to be you, for a very long time. This is the prior preparation you've already put into place that will support you being successful to the degree you will be successful. You've already begun!

One of the things I think is so great about us human beings is that we are so brilliantly sneaky in ensuring that nothing changes while we say we are trying to change. We are geniuses when it comes to rationalizing and justifying why we are doing what we do, even though there is no foundation of truth in our words or our thinking. I suspect you may be laughing right now, as you can see the humor in all the ways you lie to yourself.

Trying is Lying

Actually lying to ourselves is one of our "best friends" when it comes to staying the same. It keeps us from facing fears; and fear is the ONLY obstacle to having EVERYTHING WE WANT!

I suspect that all of you reading this are grownups. You make thousands of mature decisions every single day of the year, except when you don't want to; in which case you shift your thinking ability back to when you were a kid.

As a kid, in most ways, our parents were the boss. And in most ways, we trained ourselves to live under our parents' ways of being, doing, and thinking. At times, we were powerless, helpless, and hopeless when it came to getting them to see us as beings worthy of dignity, love, and respect. So, we found our way around our parents' authority, to do whatever we could to express our own sense of pride, dignity, and worth.

Food, for many of us, provides so much in the way of power and comfort. When we indulge our impulses to eat, we feel powerful and in control. This is a super great way to avoid feeling powerless, helpless, and hopeless. We adjust our emotional thermostat so that even with the slightest degree of restless, irritable, discontent, we head for the kitchen to get a fix of control, power, and comfort. *Thank GOD!*

So, when we consider stopping the very behavior that gives us a sense of power and control, we freak out! This makes sense, doesn't it? That kid part of us decided long ago that it had no other way to feel seen and empowered, except through this particular behavior.

What we miss when we're thinking about changing our eating habits to become more healthy, is that it's not *what we choose* that gives us power and control, it's *that we choose* that gives us power and control. So, you see, you have already started to diet like a guru, because you know how to choose to choose what you choose.

To diet like a guru, we are aware that every moment is the beginning of becoming. We are mindful of what choices align with our desired results and which choices keep us where we have been, and most likely say we don't want to be. We stretch our abilities to tell the truth - to give up lying to ourselves. We cultivate our capacity to feel our true human condition, which sometimes is the feeling of P.H.H. (Powerless, Helpless, Hopeless). And we accept when we don't have what it takes to choose differently - not yet, anyway.

One of the most elegant aspects of dieting like a guru is that if you aren't ready to choose differently, it isn't a matter of any rationalizations or justifications; it is just a matter of not being ready yet. You can let yourself off the hook. More preparation is required. No need to guilt yourself. It just isn't your time yet!

Just for today, sit with yourself, just for a few moments. With an objective perspective, notice all the ways you've prepared yourself for this leg of your spiritual journey.

Write down, if you will, the many ways you have been supporting yourself, and preparing yourself for a time when you will be taking the next step towards your desired goal. Share with yourself some of what you need to work on in order to make the next shift. Ask yourself the question: Am I ready to ask for help so I can have the life I truly want? Know that this moment of choosing to say yes, or to saying no, is one of self-honoring self-empowerment, regardless of whether you say yes or no. In this moment you have begun healing. YES!

Chapter 7
YEA FOR YOU!

I imagine that you may be experiencing a sense of empowerment and daringness today. Perhaps you are willing to look at your thoughts more regularly, and you may be experimenting with thinking differently. This is a very good thing! Acknowledge yourself for being present to this information in the way that you have been, and know this takes great daring. WHY?

We are a Culture of Neediness

Everywhere you turn you are met either by people who need something from you, or you are met by what you yourself believe you need. Everywhere you look you see advertisements and promotions making it very clear that you lack what they have to offer. Beauty, Power, Wealth, Happiness in all its different forms and colors. You lack, therefore you need.

I began this Book with Rule #1: No Deprivation Necessary. Why? Because needs arise only when you deprive yourself. Even the belief that you need to deprive yourself comes from a perception that has you think that to get what you need you need to deprive yourself of something. Around and around and around and around we go.

Because we have been raised in a culture of neediness, we learned very early in life how to distort our perceptions of truth and thus perceive ourselves as lacking, and thus needy.

To diet like a guru we come to empower ourselves to choose to decide to take a serious look at what is the absolute truth about ourselves, and what is "true," based on our consensus view of reality (aka Society's view).

When we allow ourselves to know, without a doubt, that we are a creation of eminent beauty and perfection - that we are divine love and light in-carnate - we can then practice experiencing ourselves as divine love and light, and we can then release any and all beliefs that are contrary. This cultivates truth-telling and trust in ourselves and in our higher knowing. In essence, we begin to look beyond what we see to what we know - even though we can't see it. This is a profoundly self-empowering act, in and of itself.

When I experience the absolute truth about myself, I am in a state that is perfect for realizing that I am perfect love. Whether I am fat, old, unemployed, physically disabled, unloved and incompetent in every way possible, this is a perfect situation for me to come to know myself as perfect love - because I am me, in my perfect state of being.

Quite often, I've said to myself: "When I have a husband, or when I have my children, or when I have the money, or when I ... then I will work on myself, then I will take care of myself better, then I will..."

But, few of us actually cultivate a conscious acceptance of our perfection when things are going well, because we rely on others to give us that sense of our perfection and that we need nothing. When we lose our partners, our jobs, our beauty, or our money, we go back to believing we lack and we are needy.

So each of us who sees ourselves in something other than our divine perfection are now in the most perfect place for deciding, no matter what, that we are the eternal presence of divine love. Therefore we lack nothing, we need nothing, and so, there is no need to deprive ourselves of no-thing. Whoopee!

Just for today, notice how frequently thoughts related to needs arise. Notice how frequently thoughts of deprivation arise. Consider that these thoughts are not your thoughts - they are just random thoughts that you tend to notice.

Just for today, also consider that you are absolute divine love and per-fection, as you are now - you need not change a thing. Feel into that - what is the quality of that experience, of being absolute divine love and perfec-tion? I know that, when I allow myself this experience, I'm able to breathe more deeply, feeling some relief, and that, in this moment I lack nothing, and I need do nothing to make my life better in any way.

And, if you are willing to stretch your reality just a tiny bit, begin to notice all the ways that your reality is reflecting your Divine perfection. Instantly you will see how it doesn't, because your thinking mind is attracting the thoughts its comfortable thinking (neediness & lack) You may notice just a couple or three ways at first. This is very good! The more time you spend disciplining your mind to see the good in you - the perfection in you, the quicker you will find yourself in love, rather than in lack or neediness.

Chapter 8
Try Giving Up Totally, and Completely Disregarding that You are Being Totally and Completely Disregarded

Children Should be Seen and Not Heard. As kids we are often disregarded, in regards to our being, our feelings, and our presence. Based on the experience of being disregarded, quite often we decide that there is something about us that is making that happen. We might say to ourselves: "I must not be smart enough, clever enough, cute enough, funny enough... to warrant some attention. I guess I'm not enough, and should anticipate that I will always be treated this way." Then we carry that into adulthood, and when we are with people who disregard us, we come to expect it, and think it is normal that we are being ignored or disregarded.

At the same time that we are being disregarded, we experience a violation to our essential self. It hurts to be ignored and disregarded. So we numb the hurting with anything that works, such as foods that are comforting.

Then, when we begin a diet, and endeavor to give up comfort foods for the sake of health and well-being, we begin to remove the numbing substance from our bodies, and as a result we begin to feel physical, emotional, and spiritual pain and suffering. Ow!!!! It hurts!!

As soon as we begin changing patterns of thinking, feeling and sensing, and as we take away the foods that make us feel good, we begin exfoliating layers of emotional armoring. We begin to allow ourselves to feel our true authentic response to inattentiveness, negligence, and disregard. *Yuck - who want's to feel that stuff?*

As long as we continue to armor ourselves against emotions and body

37

sensations, and *as long as we delay empowering ourselves* to experience the genuine authentic us, we won't be able to freely choose anything other than to build up more and more layers of armoring. *How much armoring are you willing to carry around?*

As you begin to take note of experiences in your life, you may notice that you ongoingly attract the same type of people and experiences, over and over again. If you are attracting people who continually disregard you, don't have time for you, and aren't really interested in what you have to say, *it usually suggests that you yourself are in some way disregarding and neglecting you too.* Another Yuck!

As I mentioned earlier, we've trained ourselves to disregard other people's disregarding behavior. We've numbed ourselves against the pain of being ignored, *and we don't even know that we are doing this.* We don't know that we are disregarding other people's behavior that is disrespectful and perhaps condescending. Our denial mechanisms keep us safe from these types of emotional woundings, yet, (trust me on this one), it still creates wounds, which need to be healed by you, sooner or later.

We believe that safety, security and stability warrant neglecting and ignoring our true authentic response when we experience disregard. However, as I just said, sooner or later, each of us will have to get real with ourselves. Because wounding adds up to something yucky happening, which will take us into some catastrophic event. We never know what that is, but quite often it is relationship issues, or a serious health issue - diabetes, cancer, heart disease, stroke - lots of variations on the theme. It usually adds up to a chronic condition which will need ongoing treatment. Congratulations, you can no longer disregard your symptoms or your wounds. You may now be on the road to recovering you human-spirit!

To diet like a guru, we begin to notice the many ways we disregard our own thoughts and feelings, needs and wants; we bring more concentrated attention to the part of us who learned how to take it well when they were disregarded and invisible. We feel compassion for the individual within us that has been ignored by others and ignored by us. We begin to build a different relationship with ourselves - one that builds trust, respect, and authentic presence.

To diet like a guru, we can ask for forgiveness from ourselves. We accept that there may be anger, hate, and rage directed toward us, from this part of us that has been holding in all these emotions, while she or he disregarded their impact. It is a moment that can be tremendously difficult to be in - we call it the Big Fat Be-With. Through this process reconciliation can begin. You become liberated and free to love again.

Just for today, notice when you feel disregarded, on the bus, or highway, at the grocery store, at work and at home. Notice what you do when you feel disregarded or neglected. What feelings and sensations arise in that moment? Consider providing some comfort and nurturing to yourself in a way that isn't related to food or other substances. Just as an experiment, be with yourself as you wish someone would be with you - a parent, a partner or friend.

This is an opportunity to begin to be truthful with yourself, respecting that part of you - a big part of you, which needs your presence and comfort. Just notice what happens.

Chapter 9
Lead Me Not Into Temptation

The greatest temptations that we face are not the substances we crave.
The greatest temptations we face are the thoughts that say something
like: "The world sees me as lacking, and I believe that I am lacking. I
hate myself for how the world sees me, and I hate that I am powerless to
do anything about it." In other words: "I am inadequate; and sooner or
later the world is going to find out about it, and there is nothing I can do
about that!"

Our greatest temptation is to believe that these negative thoughts are true,
and more importantly, that we have no power to change these perceptions -
others' perceptions, or our own. In this case it would appear that all we can
do is follow our temptations. NOT TRUE!!!

The temptation is to believe the thought that we are alone, defenseless,
empty, and guilty. Guilty, because we believe we must have done something wrong or bad to create the world's perception of us. We decide that
we are lacking in our being, and the consequence of deciding that this is
true is that we suffer alone. We live with the guilt of our perceived inad-
equacies, and we empower ourselves to at least fill the emptiness with
something or someone. It might momentarily numb the restless, irritable,
discontent, however it doesn't nourish or comfort our inner, sweet,
innocent, child-spirit-self.

Self-hate arises, and that too we wish to squelch, and so we do, with a
substance that cannot and will not nourish our spirit: sugar, carbs, alcohol,
cigarettes, drugs, etc. YUCK!

The cause of our sickness, pain, suffering and loss, is only the tempta-
tion to continue to believe that we are disempowered, and that we will
continue to be disempowered until Hell freezes over.

41

To Diet Like a Guru, we notice our temptations to think it true that we are defenseless victims, who have no power or choice. We stop looking at ourselves as if we are a glass half-empty. We put a stake in the ground for seeing ourselves as whole, healthy *and* empowered - because we are. We practice vigilance for what we know to be true, no longer accepting that there is one shred of truth in anything other than *this* truth: that *we empower ourselves to create the reality we are currently perceiving.* If we can create this life, with this set of circumstances, just imagine what is available to us, which would have us create the exact life we want to be living. All it takes is the vigilance to see ourselves as whole - a glass that is full to the brim.

Just for today, notice those thoughts that are aligned with the beliefs that you are a loser - whatever that means to you - in pain, suffering, incompetent, an inconvenience... all of these yucky thoughts. Practice noticing the ability to be tempted to believe these are true. And practice stretching yourself to just say Stop to these temptations. Stop the practice of empowering yourself to enter into a dialog with these beliefs. Later in this book, we will empower ourselves to dialog with the part of us that wants to continue to be tempted. For now, see what occurs with the practice of stopping the dialog.

At first this will be hard work - it will take effort. It won't be much fun to sit with these negative beliefs. However, over time, you will experience what it is like to live without thoughts or feelings of fear, lack, emptiness, and guilt. Honest!

I know for myself that a guilt-free life had always been unimaginable. But I now see a light at the end of the tunnel. It is certainly worth the journey through the tunnel to know myself liberated from all the guilt I've imposed upon myself for lifetimes. I want you to know that experience of guiltlessness too!

A few years ago, I wrote a blog: The Guilt Free Diet. If you are interested, http://www.theparadigmshifts.com/the-guilt-free-diet/

Chapter 10
Engage Willingly in
Being Present to ALL That You Are

It's easy to blame the past for our current circumstances. Parents, teachers, siblings, environment, culture, religion... You name it, we can blame it - we can even blame it on the Bossa-Nova!

Perhaps those individuals and circumstances were mere triggers, which put us onto a path of hurt and wretched suffering in the past. But it is *what we are doing today,* with all of those stories about people and circumstances, that is most important to focus on.

On occasion, you may have said: "Such and Such happened to me, and so I eat, drink...." Even though what happened could have been decades ago, and became the defining moment of your life, you have an opportunity to look at the choices you are making today. Today's choices create the defining moment of your life.

EVERY TIME we point to an episode in the past, we are attempting to deny the specific strategy we are currently invested in TODAY, to keep the past in the present, and to keep from being accountable for the choice we are making right now. YUCK!

Every time we point to *him, her, or it,* every time we start our sentences with *"When I was a child,"* or, *"When I was in school,"* or, *"When I was married,"* we are about to give ourselves permission to inflict a wound upon ourselves for the umpteenth time. The initial infliction of trauma occurred only once, a long time ago. So, it's you and me - it is us, who continually remind ourselves that we were wounded. When we do this, we often re-traumatize ourselves. In our current self-inflicted wounded state, we want to feel better, and so we eat. OW!

As I write this I'm aware of how often I replay old traumas. I own it! So now, being aware of this pattern, I might be willing to choose to choose differently.

Yes, something bad happened, then. Now, in this moment, as an adult, each of us has an ability and opportunity to stop using a strategy that works to make you feel sorrow, pain, heartache, grief, and agony. It isn't working to heal the original wounding. Have you noticed that part yet?

You see, many of us are addicted to the emotional state we created many years earlier, when we were traumatized by someone or something. So many of us have been living in that state of trauma, and we do not know any other reality. And, we are in denial of this reality - we don't even know we are lying to ourselves, because we don't know!

When we consider that it's the emotional states that we are addicted to, as much as it is the substances and activities we use to soothe ourselves while in these states, we begin to look in the right direction.

To diet like a guru, we look beyond the substances. We look to that which creates the impulse to eat and drink. We notice the angst, we notice the patternings that have us grab the nearest source of comfort. This is where self-empowerment works so amazingly.

Self-empowerment supports you and me to step into creating change. *No change is actually required - just look and truly understand yourself as you are.* Change will occur and you won't even feel it! It is quite an experience!

Most diet programs look at the relationship with the food or substance of choice. 12-Step programs focus on the elements of a person's survival practices, which has them use their substances. AA, NA, SA, AL-ANON, ACOA - they are certainly getting people to look inside & take inventory of the specific beliefs, thoughts, and feelings that drive one to use. Sponsors in every 12-step program coach men and woman to get honest with themselves, so that they can empower themselves to get clean of those dynamics that limit them from living a life of serenity. I believe that these are essential steps in the right direction.

To diet like a guru, we cultivate consciousness of our thoughts and feelings. We grow and strengthen muscles of courage and clarity, so that we may willingly choose to choose to think differently about the past and our present life. When we think differently we create a different relationship with our emotional and spiritual self. We have more access to self-compassion and self-forgiveness. We surrender our fear of powerlessness, accepting that we are humans, unable to be successful every moment of our lives.

To diet like a guru, we experience humbleness, not as a weakness, but as a true aspect of being within human existence. In doing so, we can let go of all of the strategies and substances that have us live stifled, numb, and quite often emotionally paralyzed.

Just for today, notice when you allow painful thoughts and memories to enter your consciousness. Notice how you be with these painful thoughts - do you invite them in, or do you escort them quickly to the door? Ask yourself: *how do I be with my past, and to what degree do I continue to allow my past to influence how I be me today?*

All of us are influenced by our past experiences, both positive and negative. It is discerning *how* we allow ourselves to be influenced by our past that is a powerful and empowering practice. Discernment allows us to empower ourselves to change our thinking and our patterns plus our habits, so that we feel better within ourselves, because we are growing ourselves - not stifling our true essential expression of the Divine.

In case you were wondering... You are not alone! You are not sick and crazy! You are not the only one who feels the way you d! Even thinking that you are the only one who knows what it's like to feel this way could be a way that you stay married to those strategies that keep you in the holding pattern you find yourself in. When you are ready, you can reach out to any number of sources for support and assistance. I am here for you too!

Continuing to participate in this practice is preparing you for greater opportunities to know yourself fully. I'm all for self-realization, especially when it leads you to empower yourself to actively engage in practices that shift you to moments of freedom and liberation. You won't believe what an amazing experience it is, to actively liberate yourself from the self-made prison within which you've been residing.

46

Chapter 11
Be Fully Engaged and Present in this Moment

Synchronicities are not just random moments in time, where it appears as if the impossible just occurred. Synchronicity is the natural unfolding of one's reality, moment by moment. The higher the vibrational resonance of our bodies, the more frequently we align ourselves with the natural unfolding of our essential beings, and the more we experience synchronicities.

In Oneness, written by Rasha - one of my favorite quotes says: "Your highest vibrational results are always forthcoming." This quote gave me a perspective, which inevitably turned my attention away from scales and clothing sizes, and toward an indicator of change that was far greater than I imagined.

We are vibrational beings. Our bodies are vibrational beings too. As many of us have heard, the universal Law of Attraction acts like a magnet within each and every vibrational being - human and otherwise. We attract to us that to which there is a match of vibrations. We will only and always attract that which is at the same vibrational level as we are! This includes people, places, foods, circumstances and more.

As you raise your vibrational level, you automatically draw towards you a different level of reality, which at first seems quite unexpected. Over time, once you get the hang of it, you will curiously await the next expression of your unfolding at higher and higher levels of being.

Katie is a great example. We've been working together for about 4 months. Through the first few weeks of noticing how she was being with herself, her thoughts and feelings, Katie began the practice of being authentically real with herself. Uncomfortable emotions were acknowledged and expressed. At times, she felt as though her body was detoxing - she felt sick, irritable, and uncomfortable. Because we worked together on a weekly basis, Katie was getting the support and assurance she needed. She came to understand that she wasn't sick or crazy. Katie began to let go of her fears of the discomfort she had been denying and avoiding through food. She allowed her body to do what it needed to do, which was to release toxic cellular memories. This is a normal and essential process for healing and for well-being to occur. It allows the body to release what no longer serves it.

As Katie allowed this release to occur, she found that her eating habits were changing without effort. Rather than eating the whole bag of chips and all the cookies in her lap, she had a few cookies and had no interest in the chips. A few weeks later, she came into our session and announced that she gave up sugar, without any fear of deprivation.

What was happening was, as Katie was releasing dense vibrational energy, which she had carried for decades and maybe even lifetimes, her vibrational attractor field was rising spontaneously. This brought about greater desire for healthier foods, and other ways of being with emotional stress, rather than eating.

Katie continues to immerse herself in the direct experience of cultivating higher vibrational resonance within herself. In so doing she continues to empower herself to do more of the same. And, as a result, she is enjoying being far more self-empowered than ever before. Katie now experiences freedom and far more flexibility to choose how she is being with food and with herself.

For me, when my highest vibrational results are not forthcoming, as I anticipate, rather than be disappointed and frustrated, I accept that there is more for me to release from my cellular memory, my beliefs and my interpretations, which trap and suppress my authentic natural expression.

To diet like a guru, we learn to engage in every moment authentically, without fear. We allow the fullest expression of our being, regardless of any negative judgments that could come to mind. To diet like a guru, we attend to our thinking and notice how we are actually intentionally creating thoughts that make us feel sad, bad, or mad. By empowering ourselves to say *stop* to "stinking thinking," we can direct our thinking anywhere we want. For example, Heather, a very good friend of mine, has trained herself to notice when what she is thinking and feeling is not peaceful. She then chooses her thoughts based on the question: does this bring me peace? It's a very effective practice!

Just for today, notice the synchronicities that let you know you are on your right path to right-relationship with yourself. Acknowledge these sacred moments, and acknowledge yourself for continuing to participate in practices that keep you on your path.

And, just for today, acknowledge the various emotions and thoughts that are swimming around you all day long. As you engage fully in the moments of your life, just notice how you choose to address and express your thoughts and feelings. Sometimes, just saying to yourself, "I hear you," is all you need to do for now.

Acknowledging yourself and your thoughts and feelings is the first step to trusting and respecting yourself. As you progress through this process, you will see how awesome it feels to bring these practices into your life.

Chapter 12
Transformation Equals Emancipation

When we are transformed, we require no managing or coping mechanisms. There is no need to create strategies or rationalizations for doing what we do. We experience an innate knowing of what to do next, and we do it. We eat what we want to eat without overeating or gaining weight! Sounds pretty amazing, eh?

Can you imagine a life within which you let go of what doesn't work, and freely allow the natural unfolding of your essential expression to just be, moment by moment? This is what this practice offers you!

I wrote a blog a few years back called: **We Want Transformation, We Just Don't Want to Change.** If you'd like to read that blog go to: http://www.theparadigmshifts.com/we-want-transformation-we-just-dont-want-to-change/ . Suffice it to say that, to choose to choose how you are going to think about your life and how you live it, may require you to choose to change some ways that you think. This is an essential theme that is heard over and over again, not only in my work but in the teachings of all gurus of spiritual and human development.

To diet like a guru, we are fascinated and intrigued with who we are, and how we came to choose to be the way we are now. This is far more fun than navel gazing, which we believe that all gurus do. We observe the evidence that everything we do is in service to having what we desire, and, at the same time, to avoid what, to us, is undesirable. We notice that, even though we think that we are serving others, we are actually serving a desire within us to feel a certain way through our actions of serving others. We create our intentions daily to support our highest truths and desires for that day, then give up control!

To diet like a guru, the clearer we are with our values, the more likely we are to choose in service of right-relationship with ourselves, in relation to our values.

It takes courage and strength to be curious about our lives. Usually people wait until their suffering is too great; then and only then, are they willing to change. This practice, to diet like a guru, immerses us in mindful intention of living in our highest knowing, serving only our highest truths and desires.

Just for today, notice all the ways you think about what you have to do to make sure you *don't do* what you *don't* want to do. Notice the amount of energy you use in service to being vigilant about *not* letting certain things happen.

Just for today, notice where there is an easy unfolding in your life. Practice being vigilant about creating more of *that* - not less of the other. At the end of the day, notice the results of your experimenting with this noticing, and if you'd like, write down your findings. Every good scientist and researcher is doing the same as you - deciding to create an experiment, experimenting, then looking at, and reporting their findings. See what shows up for you!

Transformation is not instantaneous. We have to be mindful and present to the process - one moment at a time. You will LOVE the results - I promise you!

Chapter 13
Nourishing Your Heart and Soul

For the last few days I've been stuck. I haven't been able to write. My mind has been a blank slate when it comes to how to diet like a guru.

At the same time, I've been nudged by the Divine Universe to go outside - play with my dog Gracie, walk in the woods, clean out the fishponds, and begin to clip, lop, and cut back brush, which is getting out of hand. I have also been nudged to play the cello. Play the Cello! Really?

I love the sound of a cello, and for many years I've considered learning to play one; but only when I had the money to afford one, when I had the room to store one, when I finished all the "work" projects I have in place, and when I really, really, really knew that I was really committed to learning to play the cello.

In the middle of some deep spiritually-personal work last week, where I was questioning what to do when there is nothing to do, I heard myself say: "Well, if there is nothing to do when there is nothing to do, I guess I'll learn to play the cello." This thought surprised me - as I had created all my rationalizations for not learning to play the cello.

I shared this story with my friend Marke. His response was: "I have a cello you can borrow." Two days later, he arrives at my door with a cello in hand. Jeesh!

In the 24ft trailer that is my home, I have absolutely no room for an instrument the size of a small person; plus being in the middle of so many projects, and I wasn't ready to commit to learning to play the cello, and, and, and…. Okay, you see where this is going, eh?

Being handed a cello so effortlessly, the message was clear and obvious. I surrendered to something that was directing me towards what - I didn't quite understand. My rationalizing mind said it's just another discipline - learning to play music - what's the big deal?

I had a sense that what was showing up in my life was the Divine Universe's way of encouraging me to create more balance in my life: to have other creative outlets for beauty and love.

Yesterday - being Saturday, I planned on writing, but again, the writing didn't come - and I only write when the writing comes to me, because it never works to chase the writing. It occurred to me that perhaps, until I begin to create a relationship with my new not so little friend, the cello, my writing will not happen.

I have no doubt that most of you have experienced support, guidance, and nudges from your Divine Source. Most of us know when this is happening, yet, more often than not, we ignore these communications.

To diet like a guru, it is essential that we cultivate a relationship with our Divine Source, learning to listen and respond - even openly speaking with this aspect of Self on a regular basis - like everyday (like, every minute of every day).

Richard Unger, the renowned Hand Analyst says: "You can't make progress on your life purpose until you begin to make progress on your life lessons." Okay.... How do I do that?

To diet like a guru, we need to attend to all parts of ourselves. We need to notice those times in our lives where we put work in front of play - making life happen, instead of allowing the inspired, creative unfolding of our lives. We cultivate awareness around when and how we deny ourselves fun, play, and joy, for the sake of shoulds, deadlines, and obligations.

Because our essential nature (our spiritual nature) is love, creativity, and abounding potentiality, when we deny our truest expression of ourselves, we try to fill the void in any number of ways, including food, drugs, and unlimited distractions, which rarely fulfill our Human-Spirit. By attending to our heart's desire to create and to grow, we are actually fulfilling our life purpose. Our life lessons are usually those practices that empower us to stop doing what doesn't fill our heart's desire. Pretty simple, eh?

54

Just for today, notice where you say no to doing something that nourishes your heart. Notice where you say: "Not now, I'll do it later." Notice when you tell yourself that you don't trust that you'll get your work done if you do something that your heart is calling for. Perhaps you can practice giving yourself some time to do something inspiring and fun - maybe set a timer, if you'd like.

Here is my practice: My commitment to cutting back the brush on my property is something that I've dreaded for years, but now feel inspired to take on. My commitment is to cut back one bush a day, which adds up to perhaps 20 minutes of time. This gives me other benefits too, such as exercising my muscles, playing frisbee with Gracie, taking a break from my computer - which we know is essential to greater productivity. I'm also making progress on restoring the beauty that I experienced when the brush was absent on the mossy knolls. This little activity feeds my heart and soul. I get activity, play, beauty, restfulness, and fun.

Now for the cello!

By the way: If you wonder where I store my cello - it's in the bathtub - except when I'm taking a shower. Wa-hoo!

And to state the obvious - today I was able to write!

Chapter 14

I Can Nourish Myself and Not Hate Myself

Each of us is a rich tapestry - an interweaving of threads from many lifetimes of experience. Layers of intricate threads, colors, textures, fine and raw filaments of emotions are laid down together in a complex, exquisite pattern that only can be understood by you and you alone.

Perhaps what you see is not to your liking. Perhaps you wish that what you see would be different in quality of texture, hues, vibrancy, or style. You might hate it. You might feel angry and enraged with what you created. You might experience jealousy, or envy someone else's tapestry, thinking it is somehow better than yours. You might feel embarrassed, ashamed, even humiliated because you perceive your tapestry to be lacking. Perhaps you'd like to throw the whole thing out and start over from scratch.

The you that designed this tapestry is a spark of the Divine. It is the you that chose each life experience that you imagined would create the most expressive adventure you could imagine in order to bring you to your most essential self in all its glory.

You chose to undergo the worst of the worst of the worst human experiences where undeniable grief, horror, and sorrow existed. You also chose the most beautiful, magnificent moments that brought you closer to unbearable exquisiteness of being.

To diet like a guru we bring attention to all of the filaments, and notice how we have designed the interweaving of these threads. We allow ourselves to see that we ourselves have created and designed this fabric - this life. We willingly follow each thread to its original source - experiencing the essential energy which keeps each thread connected to the loom of creation. We discover and acknowledge ourselves as artists in the creation of our own designs and life patterns.

57

Memories, culture, relationships, circumstances all assist us in designing the explicit patterns that are our own unique design.

You are becoming more aware of your connection with the interwoven aspects of your being-ness. And so you value all that you've put into this masterpiece called your life. You are grateful for the ability to bring great detail and refined subtleties into this piece, and only by bringing your intentional focused attention to each fiber will you truly appreciate the incredible wisdom and inspiration that you brought to this work.

Each thought, each emotion, each physical sensation makes up the fibers that you've spun into threads, then woven into the stories that seem permanently woven into this tapestry. Though you can talk about your experience with another human being, you alone know the experience of you. You alone travel this unique one-of-a-kind adventure. You alone can mindfully come to accept the tapestry of your life as the most perfect creation possible in order for you to love you in all your existence. You alone can surrender your attachments to the idea that there was or is a better life, a better way.

This can feel like isolation, aloneness, dark nothingness. And, this too is part of the experience of you finding you in the midst of the darkness, the nothingness. This too is part of the adventure - the only place within which you realize yourself as something greater than the flat, one-dimensional being you see in the mirror, while you brush your teeth.

Looking at your life as this interweaving of beautifully self-designed filaments of existence that you put together for your eyes only, provides you with a perspective that allows you to experience the brilliance and love that you wanted to share with yourself, through this adventure.

Just for today, notice how you look at your daily life experiences. Notice your interpretations - how you language your daily experiences. How do you talk in your head about what is occurring for you? Are you seeing this moment as not enough, less than, lacking in some way?

These interpretations, too, are part of the magnificent creation of your life. In the noticing, you are able to choose how these threads of thoughts contribute to the creation of the fullest expression of your essential nature. Just through noticing, you empower yourself to choose how to weave these beliefs and perceptions into the whole of your creation.

Because you are the eternal creator of your existence, you are at absolute choice to bring into manifestation your most brilliant imaginings. And, so you have!

I can't wait to see what you have created!

Chapter 15

Let Go of the Belief that there is a Guarantee

I recently read an article about His Holiness the Dalai Lama, written by Stephan Talty. Stephan describes the life of this man - how he was taken away from his family very early in his childhood, how he had to study and meditate, and live a life that he did not choose for himself. His country, Tibet, was taken over by China and he was forced to go into exile. Now in his 80's, he has been given many awards, including the Nobel Peace Prize. Stephan says about the Dalai Lama: "He thinks like a man that is guaranteed nothing."

Reading this created a profound awakening for me, as I realized the degree to which I have believed that because I did good deeds, I loved well, studied and worked hard, I was guaranteed everything I desire and more. By reading this sentence about the Dalai Lama, *I see that my suffering is created by my disappointment that the guarantees I thought were in place, have yet to be honored.*

I have had to take a hard look at my anger and rage, my despair and sense of aloneness, and see that so much of it comes from my belief that there was a guarantee that I would have what I wanted. However, it appears that if I want serenity and well-being, I'll have to start thinking differently.

People who live in what we consider to be physically impoverished countries actually see the United States to be a 3rd world country when it comes to spiritual prosperity. They see how we have very little capacity to be happy and content with ourselves. We constantly seek stimulation and self-gratification, from external sources. Even if it is just in the form of our fantasies about a future, where we imagine gaining power, love, beauty, and financial wealth. With that, we will get all of the security and safeness we imagine, because we believe in the guarantee.

The United States has such abundance when it comes to material resources, yet we have the most unrest and violence within our homes and neighborhoods. We have huge health problems - obesity, diabetes, heart disease, mostly caused by the consumption of food. We are satisfied with our material attainments for only moments; then, we are on to the next want and desire. We have the most, yet we live in a state of "It's Not Enough."

To diet like a guru is to think differently about what we really want. We think differently in service to creating simplicity within our everyday world, whether it is within our heads, our refrigerators, our homes, or our hearts.

To diet like a guru, we notice the clutter of unnecessary items - again, in our thoughts, our living space, and our hearts. We practice releasing what no longer serves us. With mindfulness and with gratitude, we let go of what no longer belongs to us - knowing that **to release is to trust** that we have all we need right now. We lack nothing and will never lack for anything again.

To diet like a guru, is to develop trust that you are okay, and will continue to be okay without guarantees, and without having possessions, which includes people, places and things.

In the beginning of this book, rule #1 was clear - there is no deprivation required. Here, in this moment, the question arises: "What is it that I would deprive myself of, if I release 'stuff' that is taking up space, and of which I have no use for?" Think differently, for just a moment, and consider: Who would you think yourself to be without 'stuff?'

These questions stir the pot, to support the ability to think differently. Without cultivating awareness regarding the many imaginings that keep us tethered to our current reality, we haven't the capacity to think differently or to choose differently. We maintain on constant vigilance against loss and deprivation. This is a very hard way to live.

Just for today, notice your thoughts as you move through your day. Notice how often you might say: "I haven't used this or worn this in years." Or, "I wish I could let go of the thoughts in my head that clutter my thinking." Or, "I want to spend more time with myself but I feel like I can't let go of the people in my life." Or, "My time is cluttered with social media and television. I wish I had the courage to just turn off my electronics and go outside." Or, "I wish I didn't keep filling my body up with stuff it doesn't want. I'd like to experience what it would be like to stop!"

"Once I have my house, my spouse, my career, the money... Then I'll be happy and content." This isn't how it works for most of us in the Western World. **Our hands are not free to receive when we are grasping for security and safety,** always believing that what we have will be the safety net for us. To diet like a guru requires trust (rule #2) that to have what you truly desire (Serenity and Well-being in all the most splendid ways), you need to just let go of what no longer serves you, which includes the fear of lack and losing.

Just for one second, be in the Dalai Lama's shoes, experiencing the loss of family, home, country and freedom, yet live in compassion and in serenity. His Holiness says that his religion is Kindness. He surrendered his willfulness, and found himself within something greater than himself. He had to work diligently to come to where he is in peace. If he can do this, so can I?

I believe that this is what each of us is up to - to surrender our willfulness for the opportunity to experience who we are without it. It's a big practice, yes. It requires the willingness to think differently. But to take each incremental moment as a point of choice, allows us to know that it is safe to travel this spiritual path to well-being.

The guarantee to have or to not have is not the issue. The surrendering of our attachment to the guarantee, I believe, is where we will find freedom to be in a world of our own making; one that is full of love, peace and joy. For me, that is what it's all about.

Chapter 16
What is Your Unique Practice
for Staying on the Path to Wholeness?

Today, I'm returning to the topic of disregarding yourself when you are being disregarded. Why? Because disregarding, ignoring, or denying your truth is one of the most prominent triggers for your emotional eating. The bottom line is that disregarding yourself is a practice of denying yourself.

You perhaps have noticed reoccurring twinges of pain, disappointment, and sometimes suffering, when you let others influence how you be you. Each twinge, each emotional response lets you know you are about to disregard and deny your own truth. Your body is communicating something to you. Notice when you disregard these communications!

When do you allow people to influence you? More importantly, where do you allow them to influence you? Yes, you guessed it. They can only influence you in your thoughts, in your thinking minds. This is where you have imagined and fantasized about *what would happen if. . .*

We continually create fantasies, which create false perceptions and false expectations and assumptions. We live *as if* what we just made up in our heads is actually real, as opposed to realizing that *our fantasies are just hoped-for outcomes.* By the way, it is super uncomfortable for me to write this. It hurts me as much as it might hurt you to read this. OW!

Our fantasies usually include other people being a certain way, which will trigger specific feelings, thoughts, and body sensations that you'd like to avoid. Aloneness, is a big one.

My client, Matt, continually begins his sentences with, "If only..." *If only my wife would...; if only my boss would...; if only the house was...; if only the weather would...* Matt lives in a fantasy that if everyone and everything

65

was the way he wanted, his life would be peaceful and enjoyable.

I asked Matt: "What if this is as good as it gets, Matt, with your wife, your boss, your house, the weather...?" In nano-seconds, Matt's fantasies and illusions shattered. Now he has to be with *what is,* instead of *what if.* And, for at least a few moments, he found himself outside the imaginary world within his mind.

Matt looked at me, disoriented. No one has ever asked him this question before.

Once he recovered himself, he shared that, if this was as good as it gets, he'd have to be with what is, instead of hoping and imagining something better or different. He'd have to begin to be accountable for choosing to live the life he's been living; He would have to be responsible for either continuing to live with how things are now, or choose to choose differently. In this moment, Matt just put on his big-boy boxer shorts.

When we get real with what is, and begin the practice of letting go of our illusions, we put on our big people's panties, and step into the process of discerning what we want to have happen, from what is happening. We get real with the reality around us - we begin to see the degree to which we allow our thoughts, our fantasies, and make-believe world, which exists only in our heads, to dictate our actions.

This is tough work, and each of us came here to grow ourselves up - enough that we willingly take responsibility for our lives. This is a good thing. This is an essential act of human nature - to expand, grow and thrive.

To diet like a guru requires that we get real with ourselves. This takes courage and strength. Without courage and strength we deny our responsibility to live a life that is the fullest expression of our Divine Self.

What are you afraid people might find out or decide about you, if you lived according to your absolute truths, rather than living into the imaginings and fantasies that you make believe is real?

Just for today, notice when you have a choice to make and are in conflict about what to do. Ask yourself this question: *What am I afraid people will find out or decide about me if I do what feels most true in my heart?*

This question - *What are you afraid people will find out or decide about you,* points to a core belief you carry about yourself inside yourself. You are pretending you know what other people are thinking about you. You can pretend all you want, and you can choose to act according to your pretending. And, at some point you will have to get honest with yourself about what you fantasize will happen, and perhaps choose to ask yourself, "What is it I really want?"

A critical turn in my life came when I read *Conversations with God,* by Neale Donald Walsch. In the chapter on relationships it says: "When you act in *your* highest good, you are acting in *everyone's* highest good." This declaration allowed me to get clearer about what *is* in my highest good, and what I'm afraid people will find out or decide if I live in my highest good.

Again, this is big work. And, if you have come this far in this practice, you know that you may be ready to consider the possibility of taking these questions on for yourself.

You have gained courage and strength in so many ways throughout your life, to live the best life you can. Now, you can seize that courage and strength to continue to step daringly towards your own highest and truest expression of you.

I'm telling you, you really want to take these steps, because you don't need to fantasize about who you are becoming – in this moment you are becoming what you've always wanted to be - one moment at a time. Just take a real look - no more illusions about what isn't there. No need to disregard or deny YOU!

Chapter 17
Your Mind is Just the Student

This morning, as I was in the midst of my normal practice of opening to inspiration for direction of these writings, Rumi, the great Sufi mystic, came to mind. The book, *The Essential Rumi*, (Translations by Coleman Barks), is a book that should be on every bookshelf in the world; not just on bookshelves, but actually read! That's just my humble opinion. It is a book of Rumi's writings written in the 13th century. Any writing that has lasted 800 years has got to have something extraordinary to offer.

There were many poems that expressed the theme for today, but "The Guest House" seemed the most poignant. Some of you may have heard it before. It goes like this:

"This being human is a guesthouse. Every morning the new arrival. A joy, a depression, a meanness, some momentary awareness comes as an unexpected visitor.

Welcome and entertain them all! Even if they're a crowd of sorrows, who violently sweep your house empty of its furniture, still, treat each guest honorably, he may be clearing you out for some new delight.

The dark thought, the shame, the malice, meet them at the door laughing, and invite them in.

Be grateful for whoever comes, because each has been sent as a guide from beyond."

You are here to deepen your connection with the interwoven aspects of your beingness, that which gives your life definition, in the truest sense.

We have within us, already, the capacity to transcend all limitations, in all respects.

As we diet like a guru, we realize more and more regularly that we are here only to realize our fullest potential in human form. We are here to recognize limiting thoughts and beliefs, which we've carried for lifetimes. We are here to truly grok that we are already enlightened beings, experiencing our timeless sense of knowing.

Each of us can deliver ourselves to a state of enlightened living through any number of ways while in human form. Religion, career, health, parenting, nature, and more. We choose to step into direct relationship with each of these and cultivate mastery of ourselves, in relation to each one. This is where we meet moments of enlightenment.

Each moment, each body sensation, each emotion, is a guest that we have invited to our house. Perhaps you have forgotten, but they would not be present had you not first extended the invitation.

Just for today, notice your thinking mind as it attempts to banish those aspects of you who are knocking on the door, wanting to be acknowledged and welcomed. Notice your thinking mind as it attempts to control you with fear of what might happen when you escort and invite in a monster of a character, who was you, perhaps lifetimes ago.

If we relate to our guests as God-forsaken monsters, we deny that they are Divine aspects of our selves; aspects who once experienced horrendous adversity. Their ways of being have been developed as survival strategies against further trauma.

Invite these honorable aspects into your compassionate and loving home - your heart. Welcome them and integrate each of them into your life for as long as they care to stay. You will then free them from further fear, from further abandonment, from further ridicule, and from further betrayal. They will know true love and a trusting relationship will evolve, which is more enriching than you can imagine.

Chapter 18
Be Done with Those Thoughts that Interfere with Your Thriving

The good news about life is this: you will reach a saturation point for dis-appointment and suffering. You will find that moment when you know you are done! Call it hitting bottom, call it getting wise, call it finding Jesus - call it whatever you want, but know that moment will arrive.

We are like waves and swells on an ocean. We have surface activity that we are aware of, and we have deep currents of life occurring within us. As we shift our ways of seeing and being in our everyday world, we create a shift in the undercurrents, creating swells of emotions and memories rising up from beneath, changing the surface waters.

All of this undulation of life material changes our reality - without much more from us in any way than just noticing and thinking differently. As a small boat on the vast ocean of life, we only have to stay in the boat, though at times, we will want to abandon our little ships.

Ride with the tide - Go with the Flow

Saturation points arise through allowing the natural flow of what is; again noticing that the surface waters change when we open to allowing the natural ebb and flow of the tides of energies.

Just by being aware of this process, you are releasing dense, stuck, mucky stuff. By being present to this process, you witness shifts and changes that are occurring in you and around you. And, you will find yourself delighted with such occurrences. One such occurrence is finding yourself done when you are done! Truthfully, this is a moment of transformation!

To diet like a guru, when faced with moments of transformation - when done with that which no longer serves, you face an unfamiliar moment - as if you have just woken from a very long dream. Where am I - who am I? What do I do, now that I'm aware of myself here, now?

To diet like a guru, we sit in this moment that we've been working towards for eternity. Like reaching the top of Mount Everest, we take a moment to realize all that went into this achievement. It's an ***"I'VE DONE IT,"*** moment!!

There's Nothing to Do and Nowhere to Go!

This transformative moment can feel odd, disorienting, and exhilarating all at the same time.

What do you do when you have brought yourself to an incredible achievement - a dream come true - a portal from surviving to thriving? What do you do?

Of course, just be with yourself - embracing you, your courage, strength and willingness to trust you. Think about all the challenging times, when you empowered yourself to stay on the path. Give gratitude for cultivating faith in something greater within yourself, which you've allowed to be a companion and your champion.

When you are done, do nothing, until you know what to do next; do nothing until you experience inspiration to do, or to be, different. You won't have to wonder or worry about what to do - that just wastes the preciousness of this moment. Just experience the fulfillment of being you!

With this moment may come emotions - all kinds of emotions. Much like Rumi, invite in these guests of emotions - welcome them, for they too have been waiting for eternity for this moment. Your heart is big enough - expansive enough - to welcome and accommodate a myriad of guests.

This is not a huge once-in-a-lifetime event. This saturation point is one of hundreds, if not thousands of moments where you willingly empower yourself to stop being with irritations, disappointments, and suffering. These are one-in-a-thousand moments when you choose to empower yourself to say ***Enough is Enough.***

Like being in a traffic jam, sometimes you just choose to get off the highway, just to relieve yourself of the endless nonstop insanity of the situations in front of you. In making that choice, you find some relief. Any time you give yourself this relief is an empowering choice. And of course I'm talking about choosing to choose these choices without deprivation or indulgences.

Just for today, notice that you are close to being done. Notice in which arenas you are cultivating doneness. Just attend to the fact of the matter, without worrying about what is next. Just be with what is now.

This moment of doneness, or almost doneness, is a really good time to get support. A recovery group, a coach, a spiritual guide or therapist - you are doing so much of this work on your own. And, getting support from people who can empower you to go the distance could be what takes you to the next moment of transformation.

Just for today, breathe deep. Acknowledge all of the shifts and changes you have made for your highest well-being. Never mind what didn't get done. You are cultivating sustainability, which takes two steps forward and one step back. Over time, you'll get the hang of this transformation process.

For now, share a moment of peace with yourself.

Chapter 19
Become Conscious of
What Creates Restless, Irritable, Discontent

I find it fascinating the amount of time and energy we put into educating our minds, regarding the world around us, yet dedicate so little time educating ourselves about the world within our hearts, within our souls.

Each of us ongoingly meet adversity within contexts of power, health, money, safety, death, natural disasters, and more. For each of us, the way out of these adversities is through our hearts, not our minds. I know this goes against consensus reality, but where in the heck is consensus reality taking us anyway?

Whether it's relationships, health, or money that has been the greatest challenges, you have been being with an enormous amount of emotions, body sensations, thoughts and spiritual presence. Most of you are in a holding pattern, and use all sorts of substances to numb out the slightest restless, irritable, discontent, if you can.

There are thousands of self-help books, programs, coaches, spiritual guides and therapists who empower people to empower themselves to stop numbing out. The majority of us, however, will develop physical and emotional diseases that will inevitably do us in, because we are stubborn, and we are adamant about resisting growth, self-realization, and a fulfilling life.

Why, why, why are we so, so, so resistant to doing what will inevitably bring about joy, peace and well-being, not only for each of us personally, but for all those whom we touch?

Okay, so the primary reason is that, well, we are afraid. Afraid of what?

Most of you reading this today do not live in an environment where your physical or emotional survival is at stake. However, each of you carry the patterns of fear within your DNA and within your cellular memory. Most often, you do not use your intelligence to assess the level of real danger present. Instead, you act from these memories - these patternings; not from the truth of this moment.

We are afraid to feel the fear. We are afraid to experience the restless, irritable, discontent, which may signal some eruption of traumas from our past - even traumas from past lives, which fuel our anxiety more than any other trauma.

To diet like a guru, we understand that we are whole. We understand that our wholeness includes grief, angst, agony, despair – the whole shebang! We cultivate the ability to embrace wholeness - not just in our words, but in how we relate to ourselves - our wholeness. To diet like a guru, we accept that we are so much more than our circumstances. And, that our circumstances provide impetus to truly discern what we are resisting.

Just for today, notice resistance. Notice and perhaps write down all the times you resist exploring and experiencing your emotions, and any restless, irritable, discontent. It may be that, when you experience some level of restless, irritable, discontent, you do something to ignore, avoid, or deny the source of those sensations. Before we can bring healing to ourselves, we first need to cultivate awareness of the ways we avoid bringing healing to ourselves.

Just for today, as you notice and consider even resisting doing this exercise, seriously, ask yourself what you gain by resisting. Ask yourself how long you are willing to live a life of suffering, settling, and surviving? Ask yourself, "What is the one thing I can do, in this moment, to cultivate awareness and change in myself and my circumstances?" And, notice when you decide "Not today." No guilt required, as the time will be right when it's right, and not a moment sooner!

I have no doubt that the wholeness you will come to experience directly for yourself, will be so much more wonderful and fulfilling than you can truly imagine. Having walked this walk, having explored aspects of my wholeness that I resisted before, and continue to resist, humbly I can in all honesty act as a testament to how full you can make your life.

We all just need to practice resisting the habit of resisting. Take this practice one moment at a time, for in dieting like a guru, you will find this to be the path of least resistance.

Chapter 20
Know Your Fullest Expression through Being with Your Discomforts

I love the sensation of being inspired. I love reading quotes and poems that make me say yes. I love looking at beauty which is uplifting and inspires me too. It takes me to another level of peace, calm, relaxation. I experience a willingness to enhance my well-being, trying something new, which can feel a little scary. However, usually this lasts for moments at a time - it isn't sustainable - not yet.

One of the intentions of *Diet Like a Guru* is not only providing you with potential feelings of inspiration, but also to provide enough inspiration that you willingly take action to cultivate sustainable well-being.

For me, I thought that if I was inspired enough, an effortless response of willing change would occur, and I wouldn't have to work hard or discipline myself in any way. I would just float along with the flow; I would just look to inspiring things to make me feel good. Rarely has this turned into what I thought it would.

Nothing will change without us willingly participating and acting on our own behalf. Each of us are responsible for what our lives look like. Each of us are 100% accountable for the reality we see around us, and the reality we experience inside us.

Reading this, you may feel dire hopelessness, but the fact of the matter is, you have everything you need to create the well-being that is your birthright. Each of us just need to activate the willingness to use what we've got to serve our highest good and our highest truth.

I love watching the TV show *The Biggest Loser*. I'm inspired by the contestants and their stories. They reflect the lack of discipline and personal responsibility that got them where they are, at the beginning of the show. And, over the few months that they are at the ranch, they empower themselves to cultivate conscious awareness of what it truly takes to have a great life - one within which they can thrive; one within which they are fully willing to participate.

Each contestant comes to expect of themselves a level of presence and accountability for how they show up for themselves - everyday. They put themselves through an extreme process - highly rigorous and demanding. And we, as viewers, get to see the fruits of their labor.

To diet like a guru, we live in the truth that we must be willing to take on, as if our life depended upon it. We demand more of ourselves today than we did yesterday. Willingly, we create minute shifts, taken incrementally to strengthen our confidence, and not only trust, but also know that it can be done - one moment at a time.

This process requires total immersion, total commitment, total focus and dedication. This, while you are working your full-time job, taking care of family, and other responsibilities.

The fact is, well-being and dieting like a guru have just as much to do with being 100% accountable and responsible for what you do and how you be.

To diet like a guru, you are present to how you drive your car, how you attend to your clothes, how you speak to others, how you think. Attending to the particulars of each moment will inform you of how truthfully you are living into your desire to thrive in well-being.

Being demanding of yourself, requiring 100% accountability of yourself, doesn't mean that you beat yourself up when you are not being perfection. It doesn't mean shaming yourself or guilting yourself when you are failing to show up fully. It doesn't mean you are a bad, undeserving, incompetent, pathetic, loser-victim. It doesn't mean anything of the sort.

Being demanding of yourself only requires that you show up in your highest potential, and you notice what stops you from doing that, one moment at a time. You cultivate a practice of mindfulness in support of having what you want.

Our survival strategies have created an impenetrable field of resistance to vulnerability. It focuses on surviving, not thriving. Our essential nature - the inner guru, focuses on thriving and living in faith and trust, even when we feel vulnerable. As we dedicate ourselves to living a life of thriving, purposefully taking on the task of releasing that which limits well-being, it happens.

As I mentioned earlier, I've taken up the practice of learning the cello. I was given a cello, I've bought the strings, tuned it, and every so often, I take it out and teach myself something new. How demanding am I, in this process? Thanks for asking!

What I'm attending to is the thoughts and strategies I use to avoid taking the cello out. I notice that the same strategies I use to avoid the cello are the same strategies I use to avoid well-being in every aspect of my life. Bottom line, I resist the experience of vulnerability and failure to create perfection.

My practice, then, whether with the cello or with other aspects of my life, is to be with the vulnerability that shows up. If I'm going to succeed in being the most accomplished me, I have to willingly be with the messy, stupid, ugly, failing that happens along the way. I have to humbly accept, too, that because I'm just a human being, after all, I have defects and flaws, and inabilities, which will keep me from doing things perfectly every single time. Humility is a huge part of this diet like a guru practice.

Just for today, notice how you empower yourself to willingly give into your cravings and your fears. Notice when you say, I will start tomorrow, and willingly not. Notice how you empower yourself to use your will in service to staying the same, with no change, and how you empower yourself to use your will in service to what you say you want: transformation.

There are days when that part of me that is lazy, scared, weak and apathetic has me ignore and avoid "good" behaviors. There are other days when that part of me that is wise, strong and courageous makes strides in accomplishing what I set out to do. When I admit my defects, my weaknesses, my incompetencies and dysfunctions, I begin to accept them and me for who I am. I can let go of who I am not and who I may never be. This can bring up emotions related to grief. This is a good thing, really!

Just for today, be present to the you that is inspired to have an awesome

81

life, and, be present to the you that is terrified to expand your comfort zone - even an -inth of a degree. Feel how scared and anxious you are, and see if you can just stay with the feelings. You don't have to do anything but to willingly feel what it's like to be scared and anxious.

I don't ask you to do anything that I don't willingly do myself, so I understand what it takes to diet like a guru. Gentle love to all of us.

Chapter 21
Find Your Way to Not Only Liking Yourself but to Loving Yourself

I would guess that most of us have been betrayed by people who've declared undying love to us. In our innocence, they were wolves in sheep's clothing. In our innocence, it didn't even occur to us the possibility of any act of cruelty, violation, or deceit. Within the instant that the betrayal occurred, our whole inner reality shatters. Trust is annihilated, and what one experiences is vulnerable, weak, helplessness. What is important to understand here is that we unwittingly carry these emotional traumas in our cells and DNA for lifetimes.

I believe that we are born with PTSD - post traumatic stress disorder. Past lives, collective unconscious, ancestral patternings and other influences of our unseen Universe have all combined to create within us layers and layers of experiences which have us relate to the world with anxiety and obsessive compulsive strategies for dealing with our unacknowledged, undiagnosed PTSD. Boy – that's a lot to take in, eh?

Sometimes it seems that the best we can do is to medicate ourselves with food, drugs, alcohol, and any activity that acts as a mind-numbing substance, as well as allowing ourselves to distract ourselves from those uncomfortable body sensations, which plague us routinely.

It is only when we can see the patterns and patternings of this lifetime that we can make the connections to lives before this one - the source of so much of our angst and anguish. I find it so much easier to make sense of circumstances of this lifetime, when I can see it from a perspective that includes a bigger context.

The source of our eating, drinking and other activities that numb us out, are more often than not sourced in lifetimes before this one. Through past-life regression work, more often than not, clients will share past life experiences, which point to emotional trauma that parallels their current life. We carry with us lifetimes of survival strategies which assist us in denying our emotions. DENIAL stands for: Didn't Even Know I Am Lying.

Denial is a very powerful survival mechanism. Inevitably circumstances and events will create chinks in the armoring that denial provides, and we will come face-to-face with emotions we never even knew were there.

Unless the external world thrusts upon us circumstances from which there is no escape, few of us will choose to go seeking the source of our suffering, our angst, our depressed states of being. We just use what is in front of us to feel better in the moment.

To diet like a guru, we willingly sit in and endure the inescapable truth of this moment - whether it is unbearable beauty, or unbearable grief, we allow ourselves to live the fullest expression of what is. We teach ourselves how to acknowledge the sensations and emotions that are here now; we practice being with what is - not resisting, avoiding or denying what is. We know that by allowing without resisting, it will process itself out, and we will come through the other side, relieved and free.

To diet like a guru, we acknowledge that we are the guardian and champion for all of the aspects of being that came before. Like a parent of a child in second grade, we can see the trials and tribulations that the child endures without taking on the reality of the child in this circumstance. It wouldn't make sense to do that.

To diet like a guru, we gain perspective, maturity, and wisdom to distinguish who we are now from who we were in the past. We choose to see the event that caused us grief and heartache, separate from this moment. We choose to let go of the memories that caused us grief and heartache; we choose to allow the emotions to wash through us without attaching ourselves, and simply allow them to sweep out all the emotional clutter that has been accumulating for eons.

Just for today, notice the states of being you find yourself in. Acknowledge them. Acknowledge that you've been living as if this is your cross to bear. Allow yourself to feel into these emotions and sensations - to the degree to which you can. You are strengthening muscles of courage and endurance.

These states of being, which may be uncomfortable, may include not only 'negative' and undesired states, but also experiences of joy, prosperity, beauty, innocence, play, and creativity. Many of us believe, for whatever reason, that we shouldn't experience these positive states either.

To allow ourselves the full gamut of human emotions allows us the fullest expression of our whole selves. When we deny ourselves expression, we are practicing self-deprecation. Self-deprecation is the #1 cause of depression. And, who wants to actively create depression?

Just for today, allow yourself to consider the possibility of getting support. Engage experienced people or organizations that are so very willing to be of service and support. There is no need to suffer alone.

No one is immune to human experiences which create the full range of human emotions. Because we exist as human beings, we will be in states of being that we wish to avoid from time to time. We can't avoid it. What we can do, just for today, is to acknowledge that our human condition creates ongoing opportunities to realize who we truly are.

You are a gift of grace, love, joy, and peace. I have no doubt about that! With your grace and conviction to live in your fullest potential, you will take the steps necessary to make it so.

Chapter 22

Expand Your Personal Repertoire
So You Have Freedom to Have More

Self-Love allows immediate healing; Self-Indulgence, not so much.

Having been raised Catholic, I learned early on that a "true" spiritual life was all about sacrifice, in service to love. Jesus loved us enough that he suffered for us. He wore a crown of thorns, carried the cross, and died so that we could live without suffering or sacrifice. Somehow, we didn't get the message. Most of us live a life of suffering, settling and surviving. Sorry, Jesus.

Rarely do we see Jesus happy or laughing. Prayers and spiritual songs often speak about the joy that comes when we live a spiritual life. So, why are we never seeing a happy, joyful Jesus?

Many religions, including Buddhism, require sacrifice, denial, deprivation. The idea being that by denying ourselves our desires, we will find our true spiritual nature. Well, what the heck is our true spiritual nature? The answer: Love, joy, innocence, compassion, serenity, equanimity, abundance, grace ....

Going back to our first rule for dieting like a guru: it requires no deprivation. We need not sacrifice a single thing for our well-being. We need not suffer one moment longer.

To diet like a guru requires only the cultivation of self-discovery, through which self-love becomes accessible. Self-love requires no sacrifice. Self-love invites in prosperity and connection, while it generates love in all the right places. Self-love allows us to receive our heart's desires, for we deny ourselves nothing that is not in our highest good or highest truth. Self-love allows immediate healing.

When in the midst of some personal suffering, I'll often indulge myself in something that creates momentary comfort and distraction from discomfort. In one of the earlier videos of Diet Like a Guru, I spoke about that moment when I so wanted to numb my discomfort with food, yet in that moment I realized that no amount of food - not even my most favorites, would save me from myself. I gently patted my self on my leg, and spoke softly, "it's okay, it's okay."

This was a moment of acceptance of me, in the midst of sadness, isolation, and despair. To comfort myself with my own presence changed my dependency on food to do it for me.

I began to see that in this moment, I'm able to be present to an emotional me that I had yet to acknowledge, respect, and honor. Before this moment, I just wanted to shut her up and distract her anyway I could, so I didn't have to deal!

This process allowed me to see all the ways I live in suffering, having learned to sacrifice myself, like Jesus, for the good of others. However, I found I never got the relief I anticipated. The moment of self-acknowledgement supported the shift required to live a life that could possibly include self-love.

I have denied myself, and continue to deny myself, the experience of love. This isn't necessarily related to romantic love. It's more about a universal love that just is. I don't have to sacrifice or deny myself. I can just receive love and be love, as Jesus and Buddha, and all of the spiritual teachers who are love.

Human experiences I love include making music, being present to the beauty of this moment, and sharing the fullest expression of myself beyond my writing and coaching. I notice ways in which I distract myself from universal love that are available in my life, and ways that I'm engaged and immersed in the experience of my life. I see how very different this is from indulging myself in all the ways I can, in order to distract and avoid the full experience of this moment.

To diet like a guru, we only have to acknowledge the possibility that our lives could really be fulfilling. The how of making it so will come in time, immediately, once you choose to choose love.

Just for today, notice the ways you distract yourself from what is, in this moment, and in your life in general. Notice where you are avoiding the truth of what is, in your home, your relationships, in your work life - the things that you just don't want to deal with. Notice the pains and aches in your body, those of which you may acknowledge, while ignoring the source of your suffering. And, notice how your indulgences salve your wounds, but perhaps are not actually healing the source of your wounds.

Love and joy are our birthright. Though the images of our religions may not represent the love and joy that is inherent in living a spiritual life, I have no doubt that they are ours to experience - if we want. We just have to consider the possibility of perhaps making choices that could maybe bring about change. That's all!

As you diet like a guru, you will more and more frequently experience glimpses of self-love, self-appreciation, and the joy of uncovering your delightful presence in the world. One moment at a time, you will create fulfillment in your life. I have no doubt about it!

Chapter 23
Sustainability of Progress Takes Courage, Strength and Patience

To ask the question - *Who Am I?* - will either bring existential angst and shame, or, a realization that *I am so much more than I've pretended to be*.

I once saw a bumper sticker that said: "Don't Ask for Your Problems to be Solved for You, Ask for Courage and Strength to Solve Them for Yourself." I hated this message, though I knew it was true.

Years ago, when I asked myself, *Who Am I?*, my answer was extremely disempowering. My answer was the result of the interpretations that I had created throughout my lifetime, solely based on other people's actions and reactions toward me. As far as I could figure out, based on my perceptions, I was sick and fucked-up; I was unlovable, and unworthy of loving care. And, so, I struggled to be recognized and special, lovable and worthy. I pushed and manipulated, and more than any other strategy, I compensated for my lack by diminishing my light in the world, in service to empowering others to shine their light more brightly, because, somewhere along the way, I decided that people didn't like to be around me as a wise, radiant, creative being.

Throughout the process of writing my first book, *Self-Empowerment 101,* the question: *"Who am I to write this book?"* shamed me many times. I'd fall back into bed, debilitated by the weight of other people's opinions. Mind you, these conversations occurred only in my head.

It took courage and strength to keep writing every day. It took courage and strength to empower myself to check for the evidence of who I really was, who I'd become over 55 years; who I was as an expression of divine light and love. I wrote a blog called *Am I Worthy of My Own Expression.* It was a question that occurred to me in the midst of a dream. I realized the degree to which I would not own my worthiness, because it seemed the price would be too great to pay. However, after many years of trying to live a great life according to someone else's rules, I realized the degree to which the price is much greater for dimming my light and my radiance.

I have no doubt that most of you reading this today struggle with the question - *Who Am I?* It's challenging to accept that you are LIGHT and LOVE, and WORTHY OF YOUR OWN EXPRESSION. It is also really challenging to accept that the interpretations we created that have us live as if we are lacking in ANY way, are indeed inaccurate in every conceivable circumstance.

To diet like a guru, we choose to remember our essential nature - innocence, purity of spirit, and that we are already and always perfect love.

To diet like a guru, we take up practices that align with our absolute truths within our daily lives. We willingly live the truth of who we are, from the inside out. Every day, we lessen our dependence on what other people think about us. Every day we strengthen our core conviction - deferring ourselves to no one.

It takes courage and strength to empower yourself to reject all those interpretations you made that have you hate and loathe your life. It takes courage and strength to empower yourself to look toward sources of truth that you can trust, creating an opening for love and light to reveal itself through you.

Just for today, notice which interpretations you attend to. Notice when sparks of light shine through you, and notice how you respond to your shining. Empower yourself to exercise courage and strength to defer your truth to no one - again, much of this will be happening inside your head.

Our true nature is that we are the divine sparks of eternal love.

I believe our job here, on Earth, is to reveal our true nature to ourselves, creating the capacity to be the fullest expression of our essential nature - sustainability of which takes strength and courage, dedication and commitment. I can only imagine who you are becoming through this practice of dieting like a guru. Stay present to the divinity of your being, and you'll be radiantly delighted with your experience.

Chapter 24

Getting to Know Yourself Better
Allows You to Discover Your Own Path

Let there be peace on Earth and Let it Begin with Me.

There are valuable outcomes to participating in a silent retreat - not that I'm suggesting you partake - I'm just saying that there are many values. One in particular is that, when giving yourself some time in silence, away from normal activity, quite often it becomes obvious the degree to which the lack of peace occurs within your own mind.

Sitting in silence, perhaps for five or twenty minutes, or perhaps for five to ten days, what becomes obvious is the endless chatter - most with which we participate. We rehash conflicts from the past, we rehearse potential conflicting conversations of the future. We think about the conflicts in the world and put our own unique spin on solving the world's problems. Rarely are we in a state of mind that is still and in peace. JEESH!

When I'm sitting in silence, I hear my judgments and assessments of everyone and everything. I blame my problems, my unhappiness, my lack, and my ineptitudes on all of those people who did me wrong. "If it wasn't for them...." Right? You know what I'm talking about.

Sitting in silence, it isn't about quieting the mind. It's more about noticing how I don't really want to give up the incessant debate occurring in my head-about being right, about being wronged, and about being a poor, pathetic victim to life.

Sitting in silence is also about getting clear with priorities: Do I want peace, or do I want to be right about being wronged?

To diet like a guru, we come to decide that it is only within our own heads

93

that conflict takes place. What we do in the world is only a projection of what goes on inside our heads. To diet like a guru requires taking 100% responsibility for how I spend my time and energy in relation to cultivating peace or conflict, within my mind, and as an extension of who I am in the world.

If I want peace - in my life and in the world, I have to look at the many ways I generate the ongoing conversations in my head. I have to willingly acknowledge my attachment to being right. I have to question how my righteousness influences peace and well-being. I have to use my ability to discern the values of my thinking and speaking, and empower myself to choose, only in service to my highest truth and my highest good, if that is what I want.

To diet like a guru, we experience humility as we empower ourselves to give up ego-based beliefs, which only keeps us believing that we are too pathetic and disempowered to have anything good. I've heard it said by many people, that the only thing they have is the ability to complain and blame others for their wretched life. (I know I've felt this way on more than one occasion.)

Just for today, sit in silence - if only for a few moments at a time. Set a timer if you'd like, so you don't have to focus on how much time you are spending. Within that silence, notice thoughts of conflict and righteousness. Notice thoughts of calm peacefulness. Notice moments of stillness, when they occur.

In the practice of sitting in silence, it isn't about getting it right. It's only about giving yourself time to be present with you, and learning to be present to all that you bring to your reality - within your mind.

So many of us complain that people don't listen to us. The truth is, so few of us really sit and truly listen to ourselves. We distract, avoid, ignore and rationalize that we don't have time to sit and listen to ourselves. The excuses aren't any different than what we may have heard from parents, lovers, children or friends. It's something to think about, eh?

To live in peace, and to bring peace to the world, we must own our personal attachment to maintaining conflict. This is a universal issue - one that influences the well-being of every individual on the planet. I can practice

94

letting go of the conflict I create in my head. And as I do this, I have more capabilities to bring peace into the world.

Freedom from conflict is a personal choice that only you can empower yourself to make. Freedom to live in peace is the fruit of this practice.

Let there be peace on Earth and let it begin with me.

(Let There Be Peace on Earth - Written by Jill Jackson Miller and Sy Miller, 1955.)

Chapter 25
Hope Doesn't Replace
Empowered Engagement

So many of us blame ourselves for taking the road of least resistance. We shame and guilt ourselves for making choices that keep us entrenched in relationships, jobs, and environments that perpetuate self-abuse, self-neglect, and self-loathing.

The way that I see things, each of us comes into this lifetime with a list of To-Do's. This list of tasks represents personal learning opportunities. Every one of us has to be responsible for learning what needs to be learned, and we won't be able to move on until we complete the specific learning. We give ourselves circumstances and situations within which we have the opportunity to learn and practice. This isn't unlike an obstacle course in the armed forces, or in elementary school, where we have to learn specific skills before we can go from 2nd Grade to 3rd Grade, and so on. This is due to Karmic influences.

Here is an example:

I knew, early on, that the relationships with both of my husbands were not good for me. I wanted to leave, but something kept me in them far longer than seemed wise. Karmic patterns of energy and their influences acted like a magnetic force-field that was impenetrable by me. Until I learned the required lessons I wouldn't be able to move to the next level of living and learning.

Being a student in elementary school, I had to take responsibility for learning to read, write and do arithmetic, enough to move on to the next grade. As an adult, I got it that no one was going to do the work for me. I realized that I had to take on the responsibility for the learning required to move on to the next level of fulfillment. I saw how the magnetic forces of Karma could only be lessened by empowering myself to think and act in ways that reflected my own personal accountability. Over time, I got the learning, and over time I left my marriages. Over time I've cultivated awareness to know what I want, and, for how I'm responsible for making it come into fruition.

Karma is about accountability. In previous lifetimes, we acted according to survival needs. Quite often we used violence to get what we wanted. We also used manipulation of power and people. We harmed ourselves and others, thinking this was okay. In this lifetime, we have the capacity to distinguish the absolute truth: love thy neighbor as thy self; kindness; do no harm. Since we know these to be the truth, when we do harm to ourselves or others, we reinforce survival principles, not spiritual principles; and the Karmic Field stays strong.

However, when we live in our highest truth, and act in alignment with our highest good, the Karmic Field changes. We can observe shifts in ourselves and the world around us. We feel an ease, a freedom to empower ourselves to move effortlessly in the direction we choose. It's fun and fascinating to participate and observe ourselves in relation to Karma. Truly it is no different than enjoying the learning available in elementary school.

To diet like a guru, we take full responsibility for the way things are in this moment. We become objective about our circumstances and how we, in actuality, created them, in order to fulfill our Karmic Lessons. We begin to cultivate the use of our intelligence, rather than our survival thinking, to see how we continually contribute to maintaining life as it is. We begin to put the puzzle pieces together, seeing the bigger picture.

To diet like a guru, we become curious and empowered to investigate and experiment - one moment at a time, discovering wisdom, courage, strength, and a tenacity that will bring us to a new level of self-knowing and self-appreciation.

Karma, like personal accountability, just is. There is no bad karma or good karma, just like there is no good accountability or bad accountability. You don't get good karma points for doing good deeds. You do good deeds because you are inspired and delighted in doing good deeds. You make progress with your lessons because you want to know and experience yourself in your fullest expression. If you are attempting to make progress with yourself in order to get something other than fulfillment, it won't work. That's the nature of Karmic influence as a learning tool for living within your spiritual principles.

Just for today, notice the areas of your life where you see that you are not making progress. Look at the situation from the point of view of a problem solver. Ask yourself these questions: *What are the contributing factors that keep this situation in place? What are the obstacles in the way of this situation changing? What needs to shift in me in order for the problem to go away? What am I willing to practice in support of these shifts taking place?*

This is big work, indeed. It could be very helpful to have a thinking partner, a spiritual guide, or coach, to assist you in figuring this out. It will certainly allow the Karmic patterns to be recognized and resolved much more quickly than if they stay unaddressed.

When we include the unseen power of the Universe within which we exist, we can look at ourselves and our lives with more understanding and acceptance, with more curiosity. There's a willingness to engage with LIFE in a different way. Empowering ourselves to take small quantum leaps, we find ourselves in realms of possibility we never thought possible for ourselves. It's a wonderful experience to give yourself when you are ready to do so.

Chapter 26
Prepare Yourself for a
Better Relationship with You

Emotionality Trumps Reason, Until it Doesn't

One intention of this book is to provide you with information, stories, and ideas in such a way that you yourself begin to think for yourself. This means that inevitably you will be putting reason before those emotions and body sensations that limit your ability to have the life you want, and the well-being that supports that life.

As you've been being with these specific practices, your mind has been reasoning and discerning, rationalizing and integrating the information, according to the way you currently see the world. At the same time, you feel body sensations and emotions - some of which feel yummy, others of which feel yucky.

As we mature into adulthood we become more selective regarding what makes sense intellectually. In doing so, we become more mature in how we allow our emotional reality to influence our choice-making process, only to a point, or, only within specific contexts; while in others, we still wallow in the emotional maturity of an eight year old child, or younger.

Adult Children

Though I've used the expression "Adult Children" for many years, I never really considered what this means. I knew that I was child of alcoholic parents, and as a grown up was still carrying patterns of being which reflected the life and reality of a child with alcoholic parents.

Over time, I've realized the actual meaning of the term Adult Child to represent those of us grownups who primarily are children in adult bodies.

We use the reasoning and the emotional intelligence of very young children. We do not take responsibility for our adult lives, and we look for someone upon which we can be dependent. We choose to defer our choice-making to someone outside ourselves, or to the emotional child inside of us, who is scared and incapable of adult decision-making.

It's easy to feel like a victim. It's easy to feel like a martyr. It's easy to blame others and make them responsible for our circumstances. It's easy to feel lost, hopeless, and powerless. It's easy to use substances and activities to help distract us from what is really going on inside us.

So many individuals deny their own accountability for how their life is evolving. They continue to look for ways to opt out of participating in their life work and the unfolding process, which inevitably leads them to not fulfilling their life work and life purpose.

Most of us who use substances live in denial of the fact that we are responsible for every choice we make. For instance, my dad used to make promises while he was drinking, and then break those promises, saying that he had had two martinis, and couldn't be held accountable for what he says under the influence.

Living with this person for 18 years, I learned to trust that people are very likely to break promises, and so, I came to be cynical, distrusting, and highly suspect of people saying that they love me and are there for me. Hence two divorces.

And then, there was my mother.

My mother was depressed. She was alcoholic, married to an alcoholic, and had nine children (It's funny that I think of her as having nine children, but I don't describe my dad as having nine children.). She was also the trophy wife of a doctor, and had to show up at social events as beautiful, poised, and the epitome of grace. Inside she was depressed and unfulfilled in many ways.

She hid her depression well. Anytime she was in a mood, my dad would explain it by saying that she was going through hormonal changes. So we had to drop it, surrendering to the fact that we had no influence over the situation. We had to just wait it out.

I became a very good wait-it-out kind of person. Every significant relationship in my life has been based on me waiting it out.

This waiting it out isn't like cultivating patience. It isn't about not being attached to wanting what I want and having what I want. The consequence of all of this stuff going on in my childhood is that I learned many methods of compensating for being out of control and powerless as a child.

Living with a mother who was hiding her depression and unhappiness meant that my brothers and sisters and I each developed strategies for dealing with our feelings, thoughts, needs, and wants. We cultivated coping strategies for unacknowledged and unexpressed anxiety. We didn't know we were feeling anxiety. We didn't know what we were feeling. We just knew it wasn't a good feeling, and did whatever we could to try to not feel this.

Kids are highly sensitive to such things as anxiety and depression. It's as though there are these invisible electromagnetic fields around. We can feel them, but don't understand what they are, or what to do with them.

In my family, it felt as though there was this barrier around my mother, one that did not allow me and my siblings to get too close to her. For me, it felt as though I wasn't allowed to have my wants and needs for comfort, nurturing, or nourishment met by her. I learned that it was best not to want, not to need, not to feel my feelings, and not to think my thoughts.

My inner world was confused, disoriented, frustrated, powerless, and helpless. I was always trying something new and different in order to not make my mom upset, and just by chance, perhaps to bring a little joy to her life. And, so, I went numb, and in my teens, I became suicidal.

Reconnecting with Old Patterns of Being

Over the past few days, I've been feeling a bunch of feelings and sensations that for my whole life have been buried beneath all of my compensations and survival strategies. Quite a bit has surfaced by my own participating in Diet Like a Guru as I write it. Anger, hate, angst, loneliness, insignificance, invisibility.... I feel what I felt when I was a kid, bouncing off my mothers anti-contact vibration, along with the disappointment of broken promises from my dad. It all came to the surface.

Today, as an adult, I no longer resist these emotions and body sensations. At times, it's really uncomfortable, almost excruciating; yet I know that I've been carrying this way of being and all of these emotions around with me for decades - I just never allowed myself to consciously be with how much it sucked to be me, as a kid. I never allowed the fullest expression of me. It was too scary and seemed very dangerous.

Flushing out and purging old residual emotions brings up interesting memories and sensations. It didn't occur to me until today that this is what I'm living with every moment of my life. Every one of us is living with unacknowledged emotions, unacknowledged needs and wants, unacknowledged us.

To diet like a guru, we see our patternings, and feel feelings that sometimes feel really bad. And, rather than avoiding or ignoring these feelings and sensations, we delve in, to see what the catalyst is for that patterning. Through this process, we untangle ourselves from all of this stuff, and come to peace with ourselves.

While we diet like a guru, we find mature and wise practices to support us. While we experience emotions and physical discomforts that arise, while we flush and detoxify our emotional and energetic bodies of old and useless memories, we learn to comfort ourselves in ways that are not harmful. We spend time with people and in places that nourish and nurture us, while we release patterns of thinking and reasoning that no longer serve us.

Just for today, know that you are growing and evolving into the fullest expression of you. Sometimes it sucks, it's painful, emotional, and feels as though it will never end. But know that it will end, and you will feel better than you can imagine, in so many ways.

Know too, that you may find yourself using your most favorite go-to foods and beverages to comfort you. You may find yourself taking a day or two off work, staying in bed, or just wallowing in self-pity. This is all part of you being you. These are all ways to take care of yourself, the best you can, today.

Be compassionate and forgiving of yourself. Accept that you don't have it all together. Leave any guilt and shame out of the equation. For the fact is that this process allows you to see how you learned to feel guilt in the first place. You are learning to be the you you've always wanted to be - the you that you always knew was in you.

This is sometimes scary, sucky work. But as a grown-up adult, you are also feeling the effects of empowering yourself to do this work. You will like yourself more. You will respect yourself more, and you will find yourself more fulfilled in ways that you couldn't know by living as if you were still a child in an adult body.

As The Beatles sang: It's getting better all the time!

Chapter 27

You are Sacred and Divine
Always and Everywhere

To diet like a guru, we come to experience every aspect of life as sacred and of Divine Nature. The circumstances of this present moment, regardless of how we judge and interpret it, are sacred and are without imperfection. This includes you, and every aspect of your being.

This morning, as I read David Hawkins' book, *The Eye of the I* (2001), I initially felt sad and disappointed because I so long to experience what he describes as LIFE beyond our consensus view of reality. However, he continually emphasizes that every person and every thing is perfect, beautiful, and imbued with divinity. So, rather than interpreting my life as lacking joy and bliss, I see the potentiality of experiencing joy and bliss while being sad and disappointed.

How is it possible that I could even imagine my sadness and disappointment as blissful and as joyful as any other state of being? I get it that it's only our thinking that has us interpret ourselves and our lives as lacking, which brings about sad, mad, or bad.

One of my favorite and most helpful statements comes from *A Course in Miracles:* "Lack implies that you would be better off in a state somehow different from the one you are in" (p. 11).

What would it be like if, instead of interpreting our wounds, our situations and challenging circumstances as due to a lack of something, we chose to celebrate and luxuriate in the engagement of every emotion that passes through us? What if we experienced gratitude for Despair and Despondency? What if we wished to experience the expansiveness and the sacredness of Anger, as much as we experience the sacredness and expansiveness of Love? What would shift if we looked at the idea of Deprivation as an impossibility - that there is no way in Heaven, or in Hell, that deprivation is even possible?

To diet like a guru, we willingly open ourselves up to acknowledging the absolute truth: that all emotions are sacred in essence. It is only our interpretations of them that make them good or bad, right or wrong.

I totally get that the joy I believe I am lacking will not be experienced by me until I let go of my belief that the state of joy is absent of anything I interpret as negative. For example, I can't experience joy until I heal my grief-filled wounding. The truth is that joy-filled experience exists in the midst of experiencing my grief-filled-ness. This is totally opposite to what we are trained to believe in our consensus view of reality. However, if we willingly live in our declaration of our absolute truth, that all is sacred and divine, then this includes everything and excludes nothing.

To diet like a guru, we attend to our thoughts, beliefs, and interpretations, discerning our absolute truths from those truths we were taught relative to our families, cultures and religions. We experiment with living in our absolute truths, taking quantum leaps of faith (quantum is the distance between two points, which could be a millionth of a millimeter apart - not a huge distance at all.).

Just for today, see what it would be like if you expressed gratitude for every emotion you experienced, whether 'positive' or 'negative.' What would shift? Ask yourself: *What would I have to give up to live my life this way - if only for a moment at a time?*

This is big work, partly because it requires the consideration of deconstructing a reality based on lack. I'm challenged by this myself, so, just for today, I willingly notice when I'm living as if I lack something, and see if I can shift this, so that I can be grateful for the way that it is. Through this practice I can experience not only the Sacredness and Divinity of all that is around me, but I can also experience the Sacredness and Divinity of ME!

It all is a work in progress!

Chapter 28
Serenity is a Gift of Love
You Give to Yourself

Removing obstacles to knowing yourself requires strength and the wisdom to know that you are more than what your circumstances convey to you about you and your life.

As we near the completion of *Diet Like a Guru*, you've cultivated strength, wisdom, and the ability to know, if not to experience, a more authentic expressions of you. You realize that in every moment, you are in the state of becoming. You are expanding and growing, as every moment you find yourself transformed in some way.

You experience yourself beginning to be different: observing yourself thinking and being different, as well as doing things differently. You come to accept that endings are part of every beginning - in some ways there is no difference. Like an in-breath and an out-breath, it is just part of the completion of one cycle of life.

There is always a rationale to choosing what you choose. At this level of practice, there is no excuse for leaving any question answered with "I don't know." You always know, though you may not want to know, as that would mean that you are responsible and accountable for the reason and the rationale behind every choice you make.

To diet like a guru, it is essential that we be honest with ourselves. There is nothing wrong with admitting that you just aren't ready yet. It okay to acknowledge that you are more committed to staying safe and invulnerable than to taking a step in the direction of knowing yourself and trusting yourself one degree more.

In acknowledging that you aren't ready yet, there is no set up for failing. There is only allowing yourself to be who you are, without expectations, hopes, and dreams of who you may become. Accepting ourselves where we are, as we are, is respectful of who we are now. This is a good thing.

It takes strength to admit what is true in this moment. It takes strength to give up being different than who you are in this moment. Strength is the liberated and the controlled expression of you. You get to decide to know you as you are right now. This requires attending to your thinking; noticing and letting go of all of the "yes, but's."

I love my life. At the same time, sometimes I experience loneliness, sadness, and frustration that things are as they are. In these moments I have to ask myself, *"What am I willing to change to experience less loneliness, sadness, or frustration?"* Today, I answer this question with, *"Nothing. I am unwilling to change a thing in this moment."* I know that sadness, frustration, and loneliness come and go; they are part of the human cycle of life. They are unavoidable expressions of humanness.

To diet like a guru, there is a point when we realize that, really, there is nothing to do and nowhere to go that will have us escape the truths of being human. Sometimes it is just a big fat Be-With.

Big fat Be-With's are the realization that all we can do sometimes is to endure what is, how it is, as it is. It isn't forever, it's just in this moment that it feels like it sucks.

When we be-with what is, we allow 'what is' its fullest expression as an expression of the Divine essence that is within every particle of life; within every particle of your Being.

I find sometimes that it can be just as challenging to be with beauty, love, and belonging, as it is to be with loneliness, frustration, and sadness. Vulnerability and discomfort arise, and I stand still, allowing the beauty and the anguish of being me.

We have to cultivate our capacity to be with greater degrees of those emotions we say we want, which culminates in feelings of happiness and fulfillment. Likewise we have to cultivate our ability to be with those emotions that we have avoided for lifetimes, yet have always been with us,

110

and have, up until now, dictated what we express and how we express our humanness.

Just for today, notice the ways that you deny yourself a thought, an emotion, a way of being that feels natural to you. Notice how it feels as you deny yourself your fullest expression of you. See what those feelings are up to. What are they afraid of? What are they attempting to do for you?

Our feelings and thoughts are always up to something. Sometimes we have to be sleuth-like to find out what that could be.

Over these chapters, you have cultivated new strengths and more courage to be the essential you while discerning what isn't you. It's fun, right?

Chapter 29
Truth is Accessible
Even in the Midst of a Leap of Faith

"You Can't Always Get What You Want. But if You Try Sometime, You Might Find, You Get What You Need!" ~Rolling Stones.

The degree to which I let go of what I think I need, is the degree to which I've liberated myself to actually see the truth about my needs. And, with liberation comes an opening within me to receive what I've not yet been able to receive.

Because I'm grasping so tightly to what I want, I'm unable to open up to receiving what is already mine. Truly, this isn't just spiritual rhetoric, it's absolutely true.

My list of needs used to stretch the length of my arm. Over time, I've realized that although many of my needs have not been met, I'm still alive, and more so than ever, I live an optimal life. Go figure.

Even reducing desires and wants, along with needs, has allowed me to see how so much of my life has been about struggling and suffering because my needs, wants, and my desires have not been met. A few shifts in my belief system have been helpful to making this possible. Are you interested in knowing what they are?

First of all, I came to see that all needs are related to surviving. If we don't have water and air we will die. What else do we need to ensure that we don't die?

Second: So much of my suffering is based on my beliefs that I don't have what I want. So I ask myself: *Is my life that much worse because my wants are not fulfilled?*

How much of my energy is spent feeling bad, sad and mad because I haven't been given what I want? To what degree do I punish myself for not being able to get what I want? And, to what degree do I punish others for not giving me what I want? You will be amazed at the amount of energy we expend just in this conversation alone. It's exhausting us on so many levels.

Third, most of us assume that we would somehow be better off if we had our wants, our desires, and all of our needs fulfilled. And, that we should feel unfulfilled because we interpret our current moments as lacking what we need, want, and desire.

To diet like a guru, we let go and surrender those thoughts that have us feel bad because we aren't able to have our desires and wants fulfilled. (If you are reading this, I trust that your survival needs are taken care of.) We allow ourselves to experience moments of freedom from the oppression that our thoughts create within us. We consciously cultivate a practice of letting go of what we are afraid to lose. (Something that Yoda says.)

What we experience when we don't have what we want is something much deeper than just not having a specific person, place, or thing in our lives. Our obsessive wanting covers up these deep, raw human experiences of grief, aloneness, helplessness, powerlessness, hopelessness, and more.

When we diet like a guru we see that to get what we want provides a single moment of satisfaction; however, that single moment is quickly replaced by another want.

A client of mine, Mamey, worries about money. She wants more money so she doesn't have to worry about it. The other day, Mamey reported that she got a check in the mail. She had been anticipating the arrival of this check, however it was for a much larger sum than she expected. She reported that she was elated for a whole second and a half; after which, she began to worry again about the fact that she didn't know when the next check would be coming.

The fulfillment of Mamey's desire for more money lasted just a brief moment. Then she went back to worrying, because of her incessant desire to fill a lack that she sees will never get filled, enough.

Those who perceive and acknowledge that they have everything have no

114

needs or wants of any kind. There is no fear, no angst, no worry, no lack. It is rare to talk with people with money, power, and all the toys they want, who aren't afraid of losing it. They live to protect, defend, and secure their fortunes. They may have comfort, but rarely are they happy.

I know a lot of people who were more fearless and happy when they had less. Now that they have more they have far more fear of losing their wealth. It's fascinating!

Just for today, notice thoughts of wants, needs, and desires. Notice the emotions that accompany those wants, needs, and desires. Notice what you do - the actions you take, because of these thoughts of wants, needs, and desires, and the emotions that accompany them. Ask yourself – "To what degree do these wants, needs, and desires, and the emotions that accompany them, contribute to my eating, my drinking, and any other activity, which is not in alignment with **my highest truth and my highest good?**"

To diet like a guru, we realize the essential requirement of **accepting what we have no control over.** We allow ourselves to grieve, to feel, and to express all of the raw emotions of being with what is. We take on the practice of seeing ourselves as lacking nothing in this moment. And, no matter what the circumstance, we say to ourselves: "I lack nothing in this moment, and I am grateful for the way that it is."

The degree to which we hold onto dreams and desires for what we don't have, is the degree to which we limit our ability to open and receive. This practice takes faith, doesn't it? It is just an experiment in letting go. You can always grab hold again of your thoughts, wants, and the emotions that accompany them. It's up to you - when you are ready.

Chapter 30

Continue Connecting with Your Inner Guru, No Matter What

The other night I experienced a memory. It was an almost vague moment, when I chose to be someone that I was not.

Within the fragment of being in this memory, I recognized the moment, yet could not see clearly the story within which I chose what I chose. I could feel the necessity of this choosing, in order to stay within the construct of my community, and avoid being shunned. I felt the briefest agony of surrendering my true self for a false self. I willingly took on the persona of that false self. And the denial that overcame me seemed permanent.

Though the memory lasted just a brief second, the loss of self has lasted lifetimes. The grief, and the avoidance of grief, has been my struggle. It was an ending that never came to completion.

Every single human being is in the midst of a dilemma that is parallel to my struggle. Each of us is struggling to survive, while at the same time seeing that the only way out of surviving is to begin the practices that lead to thriving.

To diet like a guru, each of us is recovering memories of stories, of beliefs, and of interpretations of what life is. We are discerning what is truth, from what is untrue. We are distinguishing our desires from that which is the catalyst of our desires. We are coming to know ourselves as we are, not as we hoped, not as we feared we might be, and not as we are not.

These are practices that lead us to thriving. These are the practices that allow us to see how empowered we are to always choose in service to thriving and to living a life that fulfills our human spirit.

Choosing to thrive instead of to struggle is a self-empowered practice that you develop one choice-point at a time. I'm betting that you've cultivated awareness of the many ways you choose to survive; while at the same time, you see that you can choose differently, when you are ready. You will be ready when you are ready, and not a moment sooner. I guarantee it!

Each of us have come to connect more fully with our own wise inner guru. We can turn to that which is always with us, always providing sustenance for our soul and our heart's desire. You never have to doubt the existence of your inner guru. You never have to doubt that within you is the source of absolute love and constant devotion to the fulfillment of your human spirit.

Thank you for walking this path with me. Though it has been challenging, it has contributed to our lives in so many ways that aren't yet visible or knowable - not yet.

I am here for you, and look forward to hearing from you from time to time. Please let me know how you are coming along, as you *Diet Like a Guru*.

Acknowledgements

This Guru Series - to Parent, Diet and Aging Like a Guru began about two years ago, when, with the help of my dear friend Marj Franke, I began to create video blogs in service to parents in need of quick access to answers about parenting (Check out www.parentlikeaguru.com). After completing that series of Vlogs, we were inspired to talk about issues raised by every dieter, and thus was born Diet Like a Guru (www.dietlikeaguru.com). Aging Like a Guru never made it to Vlog status, but was a weekly article in Orcas Issues (www.orcasissues.com).

I'm most grateful to Marj for assisting me with patience and enthusiasm, not only by being the woman behind the camera, but by asking those questions that are asked by parent, grandparents, dieters and those of us who are aging. This series of books truly wouldn't exist without you, Marj!

Fred Franke, Marj's husband and my very good friend, read and edited so many of these blogs and vlogs. He is very picky in what he is willing to read, so I always felt honored and blessed by his willingness to read each piece that went into these books. Thank you Fred!

My support team, Ruby Hernandez who edits everything I write, and Maureen K. O'Neill, who has created and designed my covers, and formatted the past eight books - I so appreciate the clarity of presence that it takes to make words and pictures into a live, beautiful expression of being. Thank you both so very much!

Bio

Dr. Rosie focused her studies in Marriage, Family and Child Therapy in the 80's. In the 90's she focused on Spiritual Guidance and received her Ph.D. in Transpersonal Psychology. In 2000, she began integrating human/family dynamics with transpersonal and spiritual dynamics, creating and facilitating the Transformational Coaching Training Program through ITP, now Sofia University.

Dr. Rosie is considered a preeminent thought-leader in the field of Transformational Coaching. Her interests and passions have taken her from boardrooms to ashrams, all over the world, in service to supporting every individual to come into the fulfillment of their human-spirit. She has cultivated the capacity to soar alongside the most elite spiritual teachers in the world.

For more information about Dr. Rosie, visit: www.theparadigmshifts.com

More Books by Dr. Rosie Kuhn

Aging Like a Guru

Parent Like a Guru

Cultivating Spirituality in Children: 101 Ways to Make Every Child's Spirit Soar

ME: 101 Indispensable Insights I Didn't Get In Therapy

IF ONLY MY MOTHER HAD TOLD ME... (OR MAYBE I JUST WASN'T LISTENING.)

YOU KNOW YOU ARE TRANSFORMING WHEN...

DILEMMAS OF BEING IN BUSINESS

THE ABCS OF SPIRITUALITY IN BUSINESS

SELF EMPOWERMENT 101

THE UNHOLY PATH OF A RELUCTANT ADVENTURER

Please visit http://www.TheParadigmShifts.com for more information. To purchase books go to Amazon.com.

CPSIA information can be obtained
at www.ICGtesting.com
Printed in the USA
FFHW01n0443060918
48055806-51777FF

9 780990 815143